Atlas of Pain Injection Techniques

Content Strategist: *Michael Houston*
Content Development Specialist: *Poppy Garraway*
Content Coordinator: *Samuel Crowe*
Project Managers: *Anne Collett/Julie Taylor*
Design: *Stewart Larking*
Illustration Manager: *Jennifer Rose*
Illustrator: *Antbits*
Marketing Manager: *Debashis Das*

ATLAS OF PAIN INJECTION TECHNIQUES

SECOND EDITION

Therese C. O'Connor MB FFARCSI
Consultant Anesthetist, Pain Specialist
Sligo Regional Hospital
Ireland

Stephen E. Abram MD
Professor, Department of Anesthesiology
Medical College of Wisconsin
Milwaukee, WI, USA

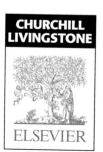

CHURCHILL
LIVINGSTONE

ELSEVIER

**Health Library
Clinical Education Centre
University Hospital of
North Staffordshire
Newcastle Road
Stoke-on-Trent ST4 6QG**

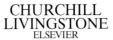

CHURCHILL
LIVINGSTONE
ELSEVIER

an imprint of Elsevier Limited

Notice

Knowledge and best practice in this field are constantly changing. As new research and experience broaden our understanding, changes in research methods, professional practices, or medical treatment may become necessary.

Practitioners and researchers must always rely on their own experience and knowledge in evaluating and using any information, methods, compounds, or experiments described herein. In using such information or methods they should be mindful of their own safety and the safety of others, including parties for whom they have a professional responsibility.

With respect to any drug or pharmaceutical products identified, readers are advised to check the most current information provided (i) on procedures featured or (ii) by the manufacturer of each product to be administered, to verify the recommended dose or formula, the method and duration of administration, and contraindications. It is the responsibility of practitioners, relying on their own experience and knowledge of their patients, to make diagnoses, to determine dosages and the best treatment for each individual patient, and to take all appropriate safety precautions.

To the fullest extent of the law, neither the Publisher nor the authors, contributors, or editors, assume any liability for any injury and/or damage to persons or property as a matter of products liability, negligence or otherwise, or from any use or operation of any methods, products, instructions, or ideas contained in the material herein.

ISBN: 9780702044717

Ebook ISBN: 9780702050343

British Library Cataloguing in Publication Data

A catalogue record of this book is available from the British Library

 your source for books,
journals and multimedia
in the health sciences

www.elsevierhealth.com

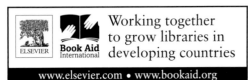

Working together
to grow libraries in
developing countries

www.elsevier.com • www.bookaid.org

The publisher's policy is to use paper manufactured from sustainable forests

Printed in China

Last digit is the print number: 9 8 7 6 5 4 3 2 1

CONTENTS

DEDICATION

For my Parents
Therese C. O'Connor
To my teachers, my colleagues, my patients and my family
Stephen Abram

ACKNOWLEDGMENT

I would like to acknowledge Florence Grehan, photographer, and the nursing staff of the Day Services Unit, Sligo Regional Hospital.

Therese C. O'Connor

PREFACE TO THE FIRST EDITION

While the role of anesthesiologists in the management of patients with severe or intractable pain has expanded dramatically in the past few decades, it has traditionally been anesthesiologists' ability to use regional anesthetic techniques both diagnostically and therapeutically that has made their contributions to pain medicine unique. This textbook emphasizes those regional anesthetic techniques that have been included in the anesthesiologist's armamentarium for many years. In recent years, there have been dramatic advances in the technology of pain management interventions. These include implantable drug delivery devices, radiofrequency and cryoanalgesia neuroablation techniques, spinal cord and peripheral nerve stimulators, percutaneous nucleoplasty, annuloplasty and vertebroplasty devices. Despite these innovations, there is still a substantial role in acute, chronic and cancer pain management for many of the older, more conventional regional anesthetic techniques.

Nerve blocks play a variety of roles in the management of pain. For acute postoperative or post-traumatic pain, they may be continued throughout the most painful interval, serving as the sole analgesic technique or as adjunctive measures, reducing the need for opioids and other systemic analgesics. For patients with chronic or cancer pain, they may provide long-term benefit by reducing nociceptive inputs to sensitized regions of the spinal cord or brain. They provide periods of antinociception that facilitate physical therapy and reconditioning. Combined with corticosteroids, they reduce neural inflammation and produce neuronal membrane stabilization. They provide diagnostic information regarding sites and mechanisms of pain. Joint and muscular injections also provide an important contribution to the diagnosis and management of chronic pain. In the cancer patient, neurolytic procedures may provide extended periods of interruption of the most active sources of nociception. Long-term infusions of local anesthetics, often combined with opioids and other analgesic agents, can provide weeks to months of relief when systemic analgesics have failed.

Our aim in embarking on the preparation of this atlas was to provide a description of many of the basic regional anesthetic tools and the common joint and muscular injections that may be of benefit to patients with persistent or severe pain. It is unusual for these procedures to be curative on their own. Their value lies in their rational use in combination with other management techniques, including, but by no means limited to, physical therapy, exercise, psychotherapy, and systemic medication. All chapters in the book have been written to a template taking the reader through each block in a consistent and easy-to-follow way. Step-by-step illustrations accompanied by photographs are used to teach technique within the context of the surrounding anatomical structures and we have also highlighted where injections can go wrong and offered advice on how to avoid problems. It is our hope that this atlas will fulfill our aim of providing a strong foundation of regional anesthetic techniques in the treatment of pain.

MECHANISMS OF PAIN TRANSMISSION—AN OVERVIEW OF ANATOMY AND PHYSIOLOGY

The term pain is used to define sensations that hurt or are unpleasant. There are, however, different types of pain. Pain following injury can be considered to have a useful protective function by rendering the injured area hypersensitive to external stimuli. Specific groups of primary sensory neurons carry stimuli defining the quality, duration and intensity of noxious stimuli from injured tissue. Their organized projections to the spinal chord or trigeminal nucleus mean that the origin of the stimuli can be precisely located. This somatic pain is often termed "ouch" pain and is usually associated with acute, direct injury to tissue. It arises from structures that are innervated by somatic nerves, e.g. muscle, skin, synovium, and periosteum. Thus the pain is usually easily localized to the distribution of the nerve supplying the injured area, and is often sharp and intense.

On the other hand, pain arising from visceral organs is poorly localized. It may be appreciated as being deep in the body, often arising from the midline, or may be referred to distant structures. The reason for this is that visceral sympathetic afferents converge on the same dorsal horn neuron as do somatic nociceptive afferents, and both of these stimuli travel to the brain via the spinothalamic pathways. Thus, pain is appreciated in the cutaneous area corresponding to the dorsal horn neuron upon which the visceral afferents converge, accompanied by allodynia and hyperalgesia in this dermatome. As a result, reflex somatic motor activity may result in the spasm of muscles. Consequently, cutaneous nociceptors may be stimulated, which may be partly responsible for referred pain. In addition, there is considerable branching of peripheral visceral afferents with resulting overlap in the territory of individual dorsal roots. Compared with somatic nociceptor fibers, only a small number of visceral afferents converge on dorsal horn neurons. This overlap, combined with convergence of visceral afferents on the dorsal horn over a wide number of segments, means that visceral pain is usually dull, vague, and very often poorly localized.

While damage to cutaneous or deep tissue is usually associated with inflammation of that tissue, neuropathic pain is significantly influenced by pathologic changes in peripheral nerve function. Thus neuropathic pain can persist long after the original injury has healed. Pathologic peripheral nerve changes include generation of spontaneous neural inputs, neuroma formation and regeneration of nerves. An injured nerve may become mechanically sensitive, and mild pressure or traction may produce bursts of rapid firing followed by many minutes of after-discharge, perceived as pain in the affected root. With time, the dorsal horn pain projection cells (wide dynamic range neurons) may attain lower thresholds and expanded receptive fields, adding to the traffic from pain fibers. The character of the pain varies and typically may be throbbing, shooting, lancinating, burning or freezing.

Recently, it has become apparent that the receptive-field properties of dorsal horn neurons are not fixed or hardwired, but can change. The reason for this is that sensory input from primary sensory fibers and interneurons onto spinal neurons is normally too low in amplitude to generate an action-potential discharge in the postsynaptic cell. A temporal or spatial summation of postsynaptic action potentials is required to exceed the threshold of the cell. The center of the receptive field usually constitutes the firing zone, where an adequate stimulus will generate an action-potential discharge in the cell. Surrounding this firing zone is the subliminal zone; a peripheral stimulus evokes a response that is subthreshold. Changes may occur in the area because an increase in excitability of a neuron can convert a previously subthreshold input into a suprathreshold response, leading to receptive-field plasticity, or central sensitization. Thus, afferent barrages of high-frequency C fiber activity can generate changes in sensory processing in the spinal cord, leading to a hyperalgesic state.

Careful investigation of the likely neurologic basis of each patient's pain may help in its treatment; thus whenever possible the following aspects should be determined: site(s), character, radiation, temporal pattern, factors increasing or decreasing pain, and associated factors. An attempt should be made to determine if the pain is somatic, visceral or neuropathic in origin, so that a rationale for treatment may be planned.

In addition, it should be remembered that there are other factors that determine an individual's level of pain perception. Psychologic factors are as important as sensory factors in determining pain perception and are more important in their contribution to suffering. Various responses to painful conditions exist, but depressive features tend to predominate in patients with chronic pain. Analysis of the patient from a psychologic perspective will provide a more thorough understanding of the patient's pain complaint and the ramifications thereof. Being attuned to psychologic issues will enable the physician to plan and execute a more comprehensive treatment plan. The relationship between depression, anxiety and pain is circular or reciprocal, rather than linear. The existence of pain often has detrimental effects on the patient's mood, increasing feelings of anxiety or depression. The development of depression or anxiety can exacerbate the experience of pain.

There have also been many reports about the perception and communication of pain, and its treatment may be influenced by sociodemographic factors. These include ethnicity and cultural background, as well as gender, age, education, and socioeconomic class.

It is therefore important to approach the management of pain bearing foremost in the mind the varying influences on perception of pain.

On the other hand, repeated blockade of sympathetic activity with local anesthetic has been shown to reduce the severity of sympathetically maintained pain. Visceral pain may also be reduced by local anesthetic blockade of visceral afferent fibers that accompany the sympathetic efferents. However, the result is short-lived if pathology remains that will cause continued stimulation; for example, carcinoma of the head of the pancreas causes pain mediated through the celiac plexus. In these cases it is reasonable to consider neurolytic visceral afferent blockade for pain relief.

It has been demonstrated that locally applied corticosteroids prevent development of ectopic discharge and suppress ongoing discharge of injured nerves. Thus in the patient with chronic nerve pain, it is reasonable to consider injection of corticosteroid at the site of injury to a nerve, e.g. epidural or nerve root injection for nerve injury due to intervertebral disc pathology.

Degeneration and inflammation of joints can produce pain that is usually somatic in character, although this may sometimes be difficult to distinguish from neuropathic pain; for example, facet joint pain may be very similar to radicular pain. Joint arthropathy as a cause of pain can be confirmed by injection of local anesthetic into the joint. Addition of corticosteroid to the local anesthetic has been shown to decrease inflammation in the joint and thereby reduce pain.

The myofascial syndrome is a very common cause of somatic pain. It is associated with marked tenderness of discrete points (trigger points) within affected muscles, and with pain that is often referred to an area some distance away. In addition, the affected areas may have the appearance of tight, ropey bands of muscle with associated autonomic changes such as vasoconstriction. Biopsies of such trigger points can show degenerative changes corresponding to the severity of pain (or can show little or no change at all). The most important aspect of the treatment of myofascial pain is to regain the length and elasticity of affected muscles. This is best achieved by physical maneuvers that stretch muscle. However, these maneuvers are often painful and may worsen muscle contraction. Therapy aimed at reducing pain and sensitivity in muscles is best instituted prior to stretching exercises. Trigger-point injections—injection of local anesthetic directly into the trigger point—can confirm the diagnosis of myofascial pain and a series of injections can markedly reduce muscle sensitivity. These injections, combined with stretching exercises, can produce significant analgesia for myofascial pain.

JOINT INJECTIONS

2

2.1 LUMBAR FACET JOINT INJECTION

Anatomy

The zygopophyseal or facet joints (Fig. 2.1.1) are paired articular surfaces between the posterior aspects of adjacent vertebrae. In the cervical region, rotation and flexion are possible as the joint surfaces lie midway between the coronal and the axial planes. Rotation is prevented in the lumbar region but flexion is possible as

the anterior portion of the lumbar facet joints lie in the coronal plane and the posterior portions in the sagittal plane. In the thoracic region, the joints' inferior and superior articular surfaces overlap each other in an almost vertical incline.

The facet joints bear most of the shear forces when the spine is flexed. In addition, when the intervertebral discs are degenerated, the facet joints carry increased load and weight, especially when the spine is extended. Innervation of the facet joints is via the medial branches of the dorsal rami of the spinal nerves. These nerves also innervate the muscles and ligaments surrounding the joints. Each medial branch divides into proximal and distal branches (Fig. 2.1.2). The proximal branch innervates the

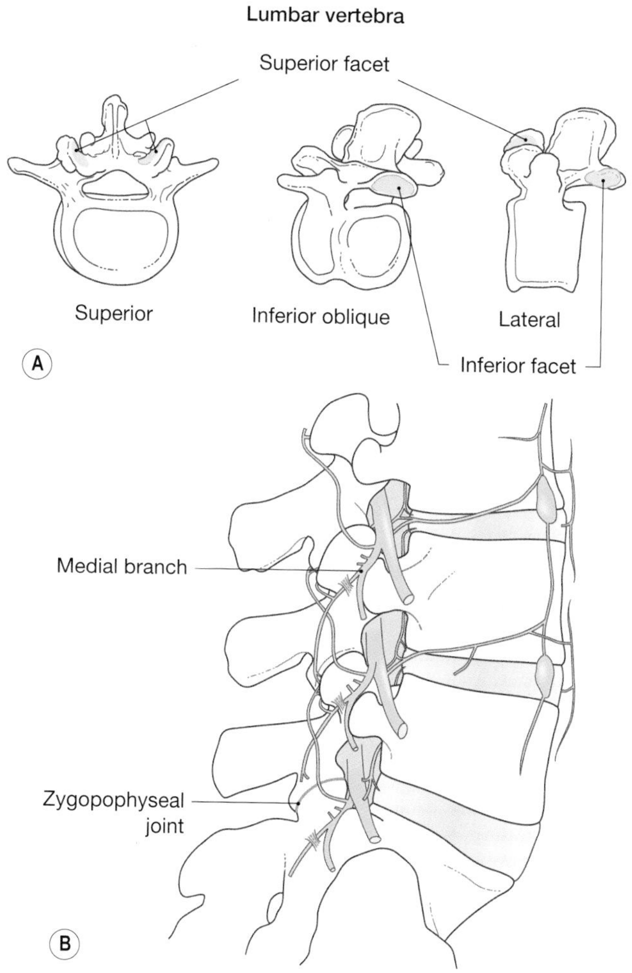

Lumbar vertebra

Superior facet

Superior Inferior oblique Lateral

Inferior facet

(A)

Medial branch

Zygopophyseal joint

(B)

Fig. 2.1.1

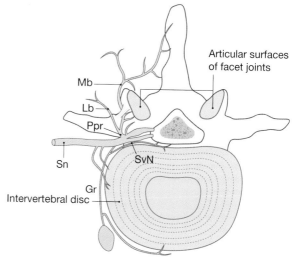

Fig. 2.1.2 Lumbar spine innervation. Innervation of the lumbar spinal structures in the transverse view. Note the posterior primary ramus (Ppr) leaving the spinal nerve (Sn) and splitting into a lateral branch (Lb) and a medial branch (Mb). The medial branch passes under the mamillo-accessory ligament to innervate the facet joint and capsule, the spinous process and the multifidus muscles. Sensory fibers traveling with the gray rami (Gr) form the sinu-vertebral nerve (SvN) and provide sensory function to the disc annulus. (Reproduced with permission from *Cousins and Bridenbaugh's Neural Blockade in Clinical Anesthesia and Management of Pain*, 4th edition, Wolters Kluwer/Lippincott Williams & Wilkins, 2009.)

adjacent facet joint, and the distal branch innervates the next facet joint below. The medial branch also innervates the interspinous ligaments and the multifidus muscles and the lateral branch innervates other adjacent muscles. Thus, pain from irritation of a joint may cause generalized sensitization of the dorsal rami with secondary hyperactivity and spasm of the innervated muscles and may be difficult to localize.

The facet joints contain vascular, highly innervated intra-articular synovial inclusions, which may become trapped and inflamed when the joint is injured, causing pain.

Equipment

- 2 ml and 10 ml syringes
- 25 G needle
- 22 G spinal needle, end-opening
- Non-ionic radio-opaque contrast medium
- ECG, BP, and SpO$_2$ monitors
- Resuscitation equipment (*see Appendix 3*)
- C-arm fluoroscopy or ultrasound

Drugs

- Lidocaine (lignocaine) 1% 10 ml (or its equivalent)
- Corticosteroid if indicated, e.g. triamcinolone diacetate 25 mg (or its equivalent)
- Resuscitation drugs (*see Appendix 3*)

Position of patient

- Prone.
- Pillow under anterior superior iliac spine to flatten the normal lumbar lordosis (*Fig. 2.1.3*).

Needle puncture and technique

- Intravenous access is inserted.
- Monitors are attached.
- Resuscitation equipment and drugs are checked and made ready for use.
- The lumbar midline and an area 10 cm × 5 cm laterally is cleaned with antiseptic solution.
- The spinous processes of the vertebrae are marked.
- **The insertion point of the needle lies 2–3 cm lateral to the cephalic end of the spinous process of the vertebra** (*Fig. 2.1.4 a,b*).
- C-arm fluoroscopy is positioned at an angle of about 30°, tilted towards the side of the joint to be injected. The angle is adjusted until the joint is well visualized. A radio-opaque object, e.g. the tip of a hemostat, is positioned over the joint and the skin is marked.
- Thereby, with the aid of fluoroscopy, the insertion point is identified.
- A skin wheal is raised and the area is infiltrated with lidocaine (lignocaine) 1%.
- A spinal needle is introduced in a **vertical direction to the skin**, until the needle is observed to enter the joint space, preferably near the lowest aspect of the joint (inferior recess). Confirmation of intra-articular placement is made by **observation of the needle tip remaining on the joint line as the fluoroscope is rotated laterally** (*Fig. 2.1.5*).
- After negative aspiration, 0.5 ml of non-ionic radio-opaque contrast medium (that is compatible with nerve tissue) is injected.
- The correct placement is indicated by outlining the joint with non-ionic radio-opaque contrast medium, visible on anteroposterior and oblique views (*Fig. 2.1.6 a,b*).

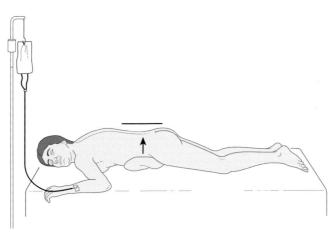

Fig. 2.1.3

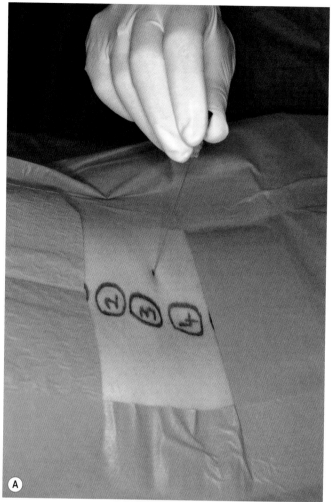

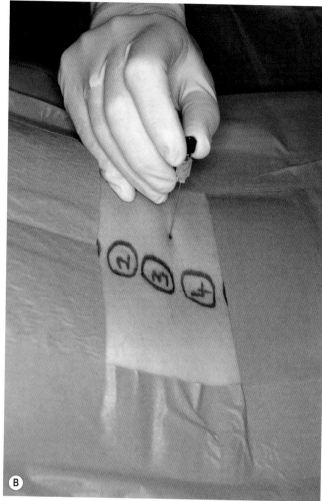

Fig. 2.1.4

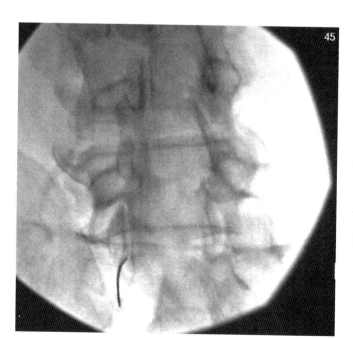

Fig. 2.1.5

Ultrasound may also be helpful in identifying the facet joint (*Fig. 2.1.7*).

- When the correct placement of the needle is confirmed, lidocaine (lignocaine) 1% 0.5 ml plus corticosteroid, e.g. triamcinolone diacetate 25 mg, may be injected and the needle removed while clearing with lidocaine (lignocaine) 1% 1 ml.

Confirmation of a successful injection

- Relief of pain.

Tips

- Care must be taken to inject only a small amount of volume as described above. A total volume of more than 1 ml may damage the joint. If the joint is disrupted anteriorly, drug may spread to the epidural space.

Potential problems

- Solution may spread to the epidural space via the anteromedial capsule.
- Nerve root injection.

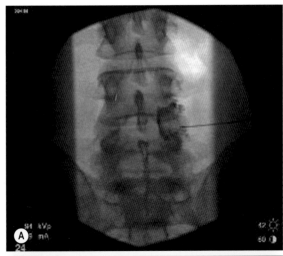

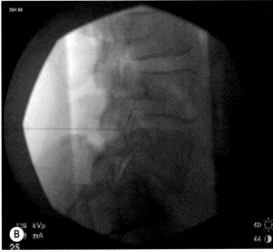

Fig. 2.1.6

Lumbar Facet Nerve Injection

- Facet nerve injection may be carried out by placing a spinal needle at the point where the superior articular and transverse processes join as the median branch passes over the cephalad edge of the transverse process (*Fig. 2.1.8*).
- The direct posterior approach should be avoided as the needle placement may be obstructed by the superior portion of the facet joint.
- Approach to the target site from a **lateral oblique angle 30° to skin** is recommended.
- The needle is advanced towards the target site (the posterior-superior edge of the transverse process) until bone is encountered.
- It is recommended that the transverse process be approached first, to determine depth.
- The needle is then repositioned medially until the lateral edge of the facet joint is reached.
- The needle is then moved superiorly until it just "falls off" the superior edge of the transverse process (*Fig. 2.1.9*).
- The optimum position is obtained by repositioning the needle to the postero-superior edge of the transverse process.
- The patient may now report reproduction of back pain.
- Injection of lidocaine (lignocaine) 1% 0.5 ml plus triamcinolone diacetate 25 mg may be carried out for therapeutic effect. Diagnostic blockade may be unreliable as anesthesia of a facet joint means that both nerves supplying the joint should be blocked. However, this means that the joint above and the joint below will also be partially blocked and therefore diagnosis of pain in a particular joint using nerve block is not feasible.

Potential problems

- The same potential problems may occur as described for lumbar facet joint injection (see above).

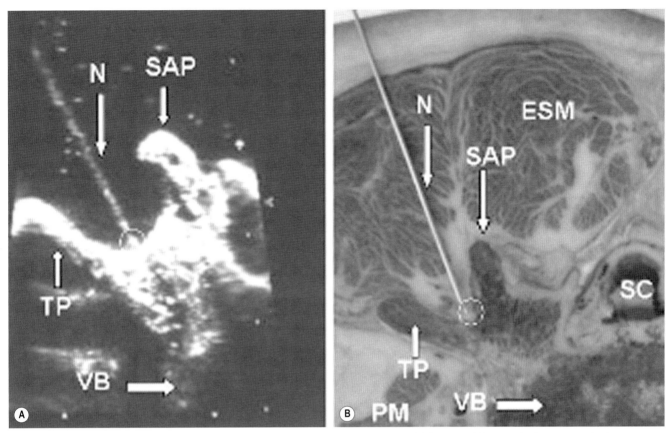

Fig. 2.1.7 A High-resolution sonogram (15-MHz linear transducer) of vertebral bone L3 immersed in water in the cross-axis view.
B Corresponding anatomic cross-sectional cadaver preparation. Circles indicate targets. ESM erector spinae muscle; N needle; PM psoas muscle; SAP superior articular process; SC spinal channel; TP transverse process; VB vertebral body. (From Greher M, Scharbert G, Kamolz LP, et al, Ultrasound-guided lumbar facet nerve block: a sonoanatomic study of a new methodologic approach. Anesthesiology 2004; 100:1242–8 © 2004 American Society of Anesthesiologists, Inc. Lippincott Williams & Wilkins, Inc.)

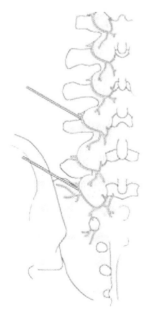

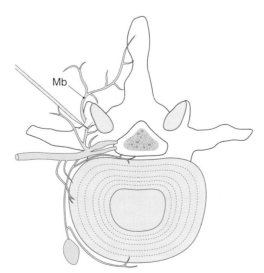

Fig. 2.1.8

Fig. 2.1.9

2.2 CERVICAL FACET JOINT INJECTION

Anatomy

The anatomy relevant to injection of the cervical facet joints is similar to that relevant to the lumbar facet joints. The cervical facet joints below the C2–3 level are innervated by the medial branches of the cervical posterior primary rami. These divide into lateral and medial branches after leaving the posterior spinal canal and the splenius capitis muscles cover the medial branch posteriorly. The medial branches lie in close proximity to the vertebral artery and the epidural space is in close proximity to the anterior joint capsule (Fig. 2.2.1). The C2–3 facet joint is innervated by the medial branch of the third occipital nerve, which travels beneath the tendonous origin of the splenius capitis muscle where it may be accessed for local anesthetic blockade (Fig. 2.2.2).

Equipment

- 2 ml and 10 ml syringes
- 25 G needle
- 22 G spinal needle, end-opening
- Radio-opaque contrast medium
- ECG, BP, and SpO$_2$ monitors
- Resuscitation equipment (*see Appendix 3*)
- C-arm fluoroscopy or ultrasound

Drugs

- Lidocaine (lignocaine) 1%, 10 ml (or its equivalent)
- Corticosteroid if indicated, e.g. triamcinolone diacetate 25 mg (or its equivalent)
- Resuscitation drugs (*see Appendix 3*)

Position of patient

- Prone.
- Neck slightly flexed (*Fig. 2.2.3*).

Needle puncture and technique

Caution: injection of 0.5–1 ml of lidocaine (lignocaine) 1% into the vertebral artery may result in immediate convulsion and/or loss of consciousness with possible cardiovascular system (CVS) collapse.

- Intravenous access is inserted.
- Monitors are attached.
- Resuscitation equipment and drugs are checked and made ready for use.
- The cervical midline and an area of 7 cm × 5 cm laterally is cleaned with antiseptic solution.
- The spinous processes are marked.

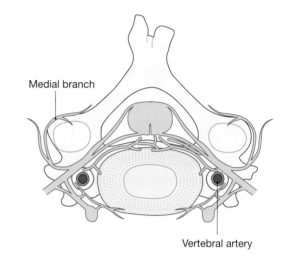

Fig. 2.2.1

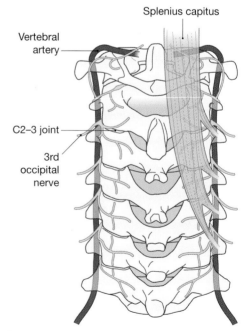

Fig. 2.2.2

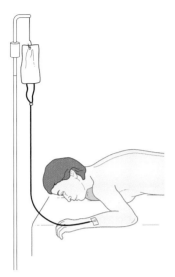

Fig. 2.2.3

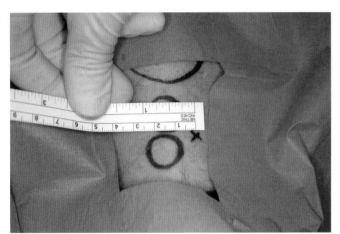

Fig. 2.2.4

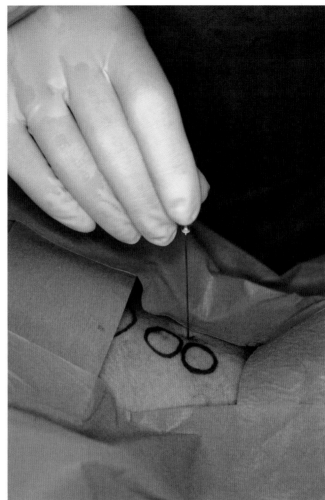

Fig. 2.2.5

- **The insertion point of the needle lies 2–3 cm lateral to the cephalic end of the spinous process of the vertebra** (*Fig. 2.2.4*).
- C-arm fluoroscopy is positioned at an angle of about 30°, tilted towards the side of the joint to be injected. The angle is adjusted until the joint is well visualized. A radio-opaque object, e.g. the tip of a hemostat, is positioned over the joint and the skin is marked.
- Thereby, with the aid of fluoroscopy, the insertion point is identified.
- A skin wheal is raised and the area is infiltrated with lidocaine (lignocaine) 1%.
- A spinal needle is introduced in a vertical direction to the skin, until the needle is observed to enter the joint space (*Fig. 2.2.5*). Confirmation of intra-articular placement is made by observation of the needle tip

remaining on the joint line as the fluoroscope is rotated (*Fig. 2.2.6*) or on ultrasound.
- After negative aspiration, 0.5 ml of non-ionic radio-opaque contrast medium (that is compatible with nerve tissue) is injected.
- The correct placement is indicated by outlining the joint with non-ionic radio-opaque contrast medium, visible on anteroposterior and oblique views.
- When the correct placement of the needle is confirmed, lidocaine (lignocaine) 1% 0.5 ml plus corticosteroid, e.g. triamcinolone diacetate 25 mg, may be injected and the needle removed while clearing with lidocaine (lignocaine) 1% 1 ml.

Confirmation of a successful injection

- Relief of pain.

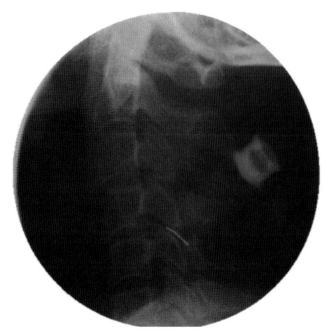

Fig. 2.2.6

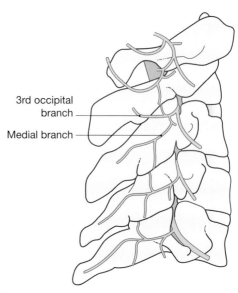

3rd occipital
branch

Medial branch

Fig. 2.2.7

Tips

- Care must be taken to inject only a small amount of volume, as described above. A total volume of more than 1 ml may damage the joint. If the joint is disrupted anteriorly, a drug may spread to the epidural space.

Potential problems

- Solution may spread to the epidural space via the anteromedial capsule.
- Nerve root injection.
- Intrathecal injection resulting in spinal anesthesia may occur if local anesthetic is inadvertently injected into the nerve root sleeve. Prompt recognition of this complication is vital during cervical procedures, because the patient's breathing may be arrested and there may be immediate convulsion and/or loss of consciousness with CVS collapse requiring immediate resuscitation. In addition, the patient's head should be immediately elevated after the injection to ensure that the lidocaine (lignocaine) flows inferiorly. Some practitioners elevate the head of the table during all cervical injections to help prevent this complication. Intravenous injection may be harmless, but it results in a suboptimal or false-negative result.
- Intra-arterial injection may result in immediate convulsion and/or loss of consciousness with possible CVS collapse. Intrarterial injection can be dangerous if the agent is injected into the vertebral artery or radicular branches that enter the neural foramina at various levels

and, rarely, persisting paraplegia or paraparesis have been reported after cervical facet joint injection or nerve root block. These complications may be due to embolism from intra-arterial injection of particulate corticosteroid. However, even when contrast injection prior to steroid infiltration confirms extravascular needle placement, nerve damage may occur, which suggests an alternative cause for the complication, such as vasospasm or direct arterial injury from the needle-tip. Regardless of the cause, contrast injection is recommended to at least potentially reduce the risk of intravascular injection. Ultrasound will have limitations in this regard.
- Hematoma may occur (avoid performing block on patients who have coagulopathy).

CERVICAL FACET NERVE INJECTION

- Facet nerve injection may be carried out by placing a spinal needle at the point where the superior articular and transverse processes join as the median branch passes over the cephalad edge of the transverse process (*Fig. 2.2.7*).
- The direct posterior approach should be avoided as the needle placement may be obstructed by the superior portion of the facet joint.
- Approach to the target site from a **lateral oblique angle 30° to the skin** is recommended.
- The needle is advanced towards the target site (the posterior–superior edge of the transverse process) until bone is encountered.
- It is recommended that the transverse process be approached first, to determine depth.

- The needle is then repositioned medially until the lateral edge of the facet joint is reached.
- The needle is then moved superiorly until it just "falls off" the superior edge of the transverse process.
- The optimum position is obtained by repositioning the needle to the posterosuperior edge of the transverse process.
- The patient may now report reproduction of back pain.

- Injection of lidocaine (lignocaine) 1% 0.5 ml plus triamcinolone diacetate 25 mg may be carried out for therapeutic effect. Diagnostic blockade may be unreliable as anesthesia of a facet joint means that both nerves supplying the joint should be blocked. However, this means that the joint above and the joint below will also be partially blocked and therefore diagnosis of pain in a particular joint using nerve block is not feasible.

2.3 SACRO-ILIAC JOINT INJECTION

Anatomy

The surfaces of the sacrum and ilium form a synovial joint, the sacro-iliac joint. Ligaments and connective tissue surround the joint, conferring stability and preventing excessive movement of the joint (Figs 2.3.1, 2.3.2). The joint is innervated by L4, L5, S1 (the superior gluteal nerve), S2, and L3. Localization of the pain is therefore difficult due to this wide nerve supply to the joint.

Equipment

- 2 ml and 10 ml syringes
- 25 G needle

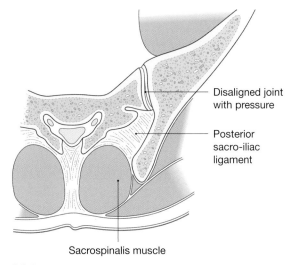

Disaligned joint with pressure

Posterior sacro-iliac ligament

Sacrospinalis muscle

Fig. 2.3.1

- 22 G spinal needle, end-opening
- Radio-opaque contrast medium
- ECG, BP, and SpO$_2$ monitors
- Resuscitation equipment (*see Appendix 3*)
- C-arm fluoroscopy or ultrasound

Drugs

- Lidocaine (lignocaine) 1%, 10 ml (or its equivalent)
- Corticosteroid if indicated, e.g. triamcinolone diacetate 25 mg (or its equivalent)
- Resuscitation drugs (*see Appendix 3*)

Position of patient

- Prone.
- Pillow under anterior superior iliac spine to flatten the normal lumbar lordosis (*Fig. 2.3.3*).

Needle puncture and technique

- Intravenous access is inserted.
- Monitors are attached.
- Resuscitation equipment and drugs are checked and made ready for use.
- The sacral area is prepared antiseptically.
- An AP image is obtained, centered over the joint to be injected.
- Two joint lines are observed. The posterior joint line is located more medial in a direct AP view (*Fig. 2.3.4a*). The image intensifier (positioned above the patient) is rotated toward the opposite side until the two joint lines

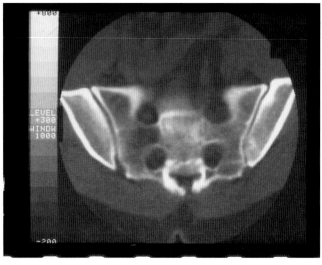

Fig. 2.3.2

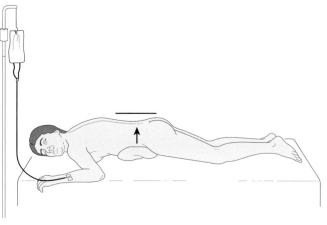

Fig. 2.3.3

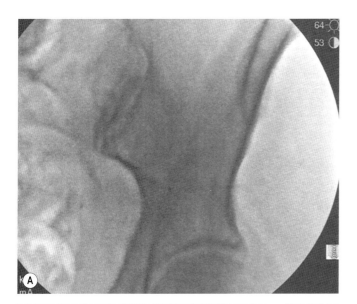

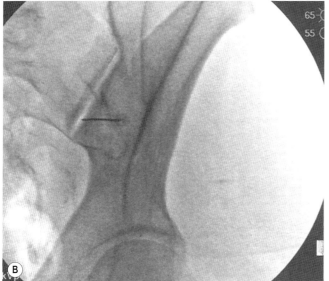

Fig. 2.3.4

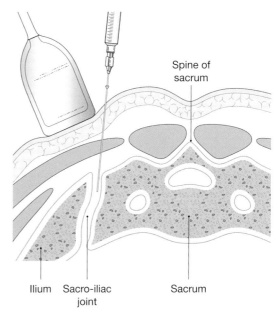

Spine of
sacrum

Ilium   Sacro-iliac   Sacrum
              joint

Fig. 2.3.5

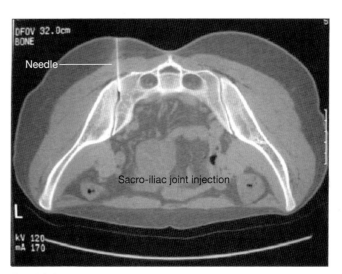

DFOV 32.0cm
BONE

Needle

Sacro-iliac joint injection

L

kV 120
mA 170

Fig. 2.3.6

are superimposed (usually about 10–20°) (*Fig. 2.3.4b*). The skin is marked and a skin wheal is raised. The area is infiltrated with lidocaine (lignocaine) 1% **over the joint line 1 cm above the most caudal point of the joint.**

- A 22 or 25 G 3½ in spinal needle is advanced no more than 1 cm into the joint. Some resistance is usually felt as the needle contacts the joint.
- A lateral view is then obtained. The needle should traverse no more than half the distance across the sacrum, and should never be advanced beyond the anterior cortex.
- Contrast dye, 0.5 to 1 ml, may be injected to ensure intra-articular spread. Intravascular injection is best detected during "live" fluoroscopy injection. In the AP view, dye should be seen within the joint space. Some

extravasation outside the joint is common. If extensive, the needle should be repositioned.

- 1–2 ml lidocaine 1% is injected alone for diagnostic purposes. Reproduction of the patient's pain during needle positioning and injection as well as pain relief following the block will help confirm the sacro-iliac joint as the pain generator (avoid sedation with opioids for diagnostic procedures).
- Corticosteroid, e.g. triamcinolone diacetate 25 mg, plus 1–2 ml 1% lidocaine may be injected for therapeutic effect.
- Ultrasound may also be used to identify the joint (*Fig. 2.3.5*).
- CT scan may also be used to identify the joint but is not usually necessary (*Fig. 2.3.6*).

Confirmation of a successful injection

- Reproduction of pain during injection and relief of pain following injection confirms correct placement.
- Radiologic assessment of the X-ray image after injection of contrast medium may demonstrate tears in the joint capsule.

Tips

- While the joint may be easily entered, injection can be difficult where the joint is heavily invested with connective tissue and ligaments. This is especially true in elderly patients, where the joint is rigid and the joint space cannot expand to accommodate a volume of liquid. In such cases it may be possible to inject only as the needle is being removed from the joint.

- Sometimes, injection into the deep sacro-iliac ligaments around the joint may be helpful for pain relief. Introduction of a spinal needle just above the midline of the upper sacrum and advanced at 45° to the skin, under the rim of the ilium and in the direction of the joint, will access these ligaments. Lidocaine (lignocaine) 1% 4 ml plus triamcinolone diacetate 25 mg may then be injected.

Potential problems

- Discomfort on injection.
- Epidural injection.
- Sacral nerve root blockade.
- Subperiosteal injection (painful in the awake patient).

EPIDURAL INJECTION

Intervertebral disc disease may produce inflammation of spinal nerve roots, which may be the cause of radicular pain. The L5 and S1 nerve roots are most commonly affected, probably because they exit the bony canal through a narrow lateral bony recess, therefore increasing the likelihood of nerve compression and irritation. Lumbo-sacral radiculopathy consists of low-back pain that radiates a varying distance into the lower extremity, and which may be associated with motor and sensory loss consistent with damage to the affected nerve root. If bowel and bladder symptoms of dysfunction are present, large midline disc protrusion is suspected and prompt surgical intervention is indicated. Otherwise, if severe pain exists after treatment with immobilization and mild analgesics, epidural steroid injection may be carried out. Similarly, pain of thoracic or cervical disc origin may respond to epidural steroid injection.

Triamcinolone diacetate is the most commonly administered preparation and injection should be carried out as close to the affected nerve root as possible. Injection of a small amount of local anesthetic with the steroid will help to confirm drug placement and provide analgesia. In patients with S1 pathology the drug may not spread to the affected nerve root using the lumbar approach and the caudal approach to the epidural space may be required. Cervical epidural injection accesses the cervical spinal nerve roots, while in the thoracic region a paramedian approach is usually more successful.

3.1 LUMBAR EPIDURAL BLOCK

Anatomy

Structures encountered when inserting an epidural needle include skin, subcutaneous tissue, supraspinous ligament, interspinous ligament, ligamentum flavum (5–6 mm thick in the midline of the lumbar region, 3–5 mm thick in the midline of the thoracic region), prior to reaching the epidural space itself (Fig. 3.1.1). Beyond this space lies the dura mater, the arachnoid mater and intrathecal space containing the cerebrospinal fluid. The spinal cord usually ends at the L2 level (Fig. 3.1.2).

One should expect a distance of 3.5–6 cm from skin to the epidural space using a midline approach. In the lumbar region the spinous processes are generally perpendicular to the vertebral bodies (Fig. 3.1.3). In the thoracic region the spinous processes lie at an angle of 30–45° to the thoracic vertebral body, thus making midline epidural injection a little more difficult, and sometimes necessitating a paravertebral approach. Other relevant anatomy of the vertebral bodies is illustrated in Fig. 3.1.4.

Equipment

- 2 ml and 10 ml syringes
- 18 G, 20 G, and 25 G needles
- ECG, BP, and SpO_2 monitors
- 18 G epidural set (*Fig. 3.1.5*)
- Filter aspiration needle
- Resuscitation equipment (*see Appendix 3*)
- Fluoroscopy (optional)
- Ultrasound (optional)

Drugs

- Lidocaine (lignocaine) 1%, 10 ml (or its equivalent)
- Corticosteroid if indicated, e.g. triamcinolone diacetate 50 mg (or its equivalent)
- Saline (NaCl) 10 ml
- Resuscitation drugs (*see Appendix 3*)

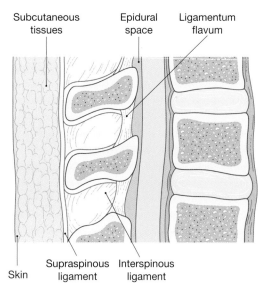

Fig. 3.1.1

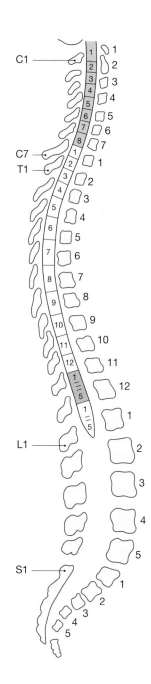

Fig. 3.1.2

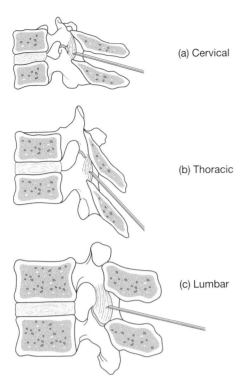

Fig. 3.1.3

Position of patient

- Lateral, usually lying on the side of the radiculopathy.
- Shoulders and buttocks parallel to the edge of the bed, perpendicular to the floor, with spine flexed.

Needle puncture and technique

- Intravenous access is inserted.
- Monitors are attached.
- Resuscitation equipment and drugs are checked and made ready for use.
- The midline and an area 10 cm × 5 cm laterally is cleaned with antiseptic solution and a fenestrated drape is placed over the sterile area.
- Lidocaine (lignocaine) 1% 2 ml is drawn up into three 2 ml syringes.
- Lidocaine (lignocaine) 1% 2 ml, plus corticosteroid, e.g. triamcinolone diacetate 50 mg is drawn up into the 10 ml syringe.
- NaCl 10 ml is drawn up into the 10 ml loss-of-resistance syringe.
- The iliac crest is palpated and the intercrestal line (this corresponds with the inferior aspect of the spinous process of L4 or may lie in the L4–5 interspace) is identified (*Fig. 3.1.6*).
- The spinous processes are palpated, and the level requiring injection is identified.
- This may be confirmed by fluoroscopy or ultrasound.

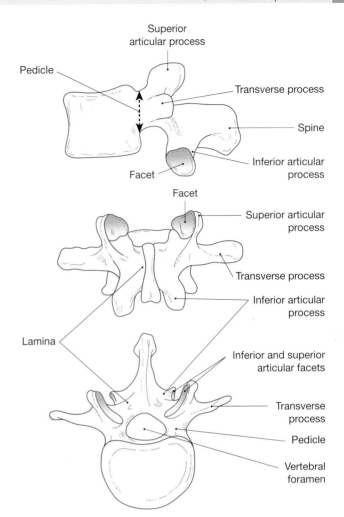

Fig. 3.1.4

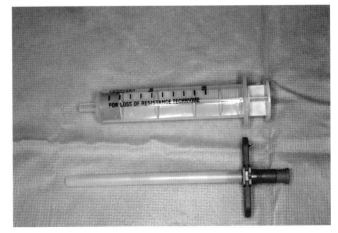

Fig. 3.1.5

MIDLINE APPROACH FOR THE RIGHT-HANDED OPERATOR

With the left hand
- The fore- and middle fingers are placed each side of the interspace.

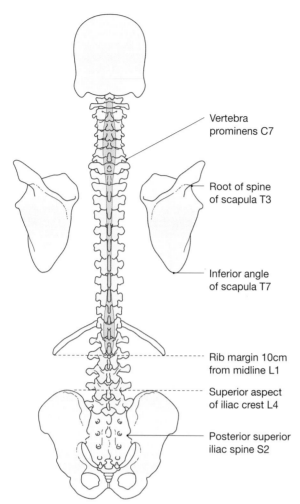

Fig. 3.1.6

Vertebra
prominens C7

Root of spine
of scapula T3

Inferior angle
of scapula T7

Rib margin 10cm
from midline L1

Superior aspect
of iliac crest L4

Posterior superior
iliac spine S2

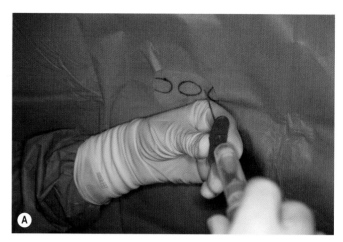

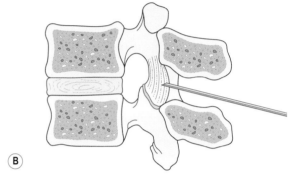

Fig. 3.1.7

- These fingers are kept in place until the epidural needle is gripped by the interspinous ligament.

With the right hand
- The interspinous ligament is infiltrated with lidocaine (lignocaine) 1% 2 ml.
- **The epidural needle is inserted, bevel facing the side of the radiculopathy, between the fore- and middle fingers of the left hand in a direction 60° cephalad, perpendicular to the spine, parallel to the floor, until it is gripped by the interspinous ligament** (*Fig. 3.1.7 a,b*). In the case of thoracic epidural injection (midline approach), the point of entry of the needle should be as close as possible to the caudal end of the interspinous space and the needle directed 30–45° cephalad to enter between the spinous processes.
- The hub of the needle is gripped with the fore- and middle fingers of the left hand and this hand is steadied by leaning the wrist against the patient's back.
- The stylet is removed and the loss-of-resistance syringe is applied.

- The needle is slowly and carefully advanced, while constant pressure is applied to the plunger, the left hand aiding the advance, while at the same time applying a brake if required (*Fig. 3.1.8 a,b*).
- At the point at which the needle enters the ligamentum flavum, absolute resistance to injection is experienced.
- At this point the needle is advanced very slowly until a sudden loss of resistance to the pressure on the plunger is experienced, the point at which the epidural space is entered.
- After negative aspiration for blood or cerebrospinal fluid (CSF), lidocaine (lignocaine) 1% 3 ml is injected.
- After 5 minutes the patient is questioned about any changes in sensation or power, and any changes in heart rate or blood pressure are noted.
- If the injection is for diagnostic purposes only, the needle may be removed at this point.
- If therapeutic effect is required, lidocaine (lignocaine) 1% 2 ml, plus corticosteroid if indicated, e.g. triamcinolone diacetate 50 mg (or its equivalent), may be injected. Alternatively, a catheter may be inserted through the needle if indicated.
- The needle is flushed with NaCl 1 ml and removed.
- The patient is allowed to lie in the lateral position, on the side of the pain.

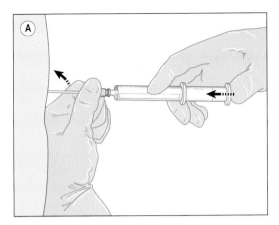

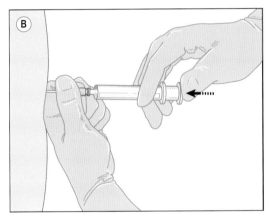

Fig. 3.1.8

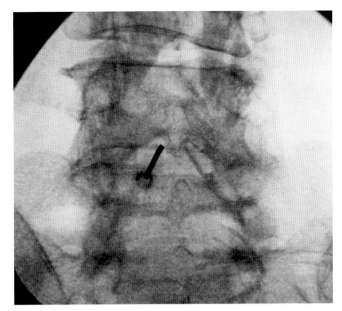

Fig. 3.1.9

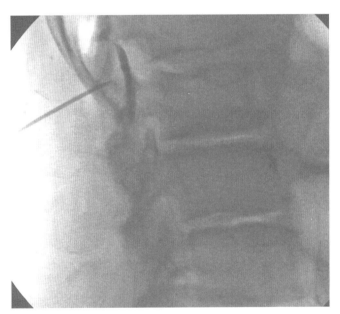

Fig. 3.1.10

- Monitors should be left attached and i.v. access left in situ for at least 30 minutes.
- The patient is advised to contact the hospital should the anesthesia remain after several hours.

FLUOROSCOPIC GUIDED LUMBAR EPIDURAL INJECTION

- Position the patient prone with a pillow under the lower abdomen to increase lumbar flexion.
- The interlaminar space for the desired segmental level is identified fluoroscopically using a straight AP view. Angling the fluoroscope slightly cephalad may open the space if it appears very narrow.
- Prepare skin with antiseptic and sterile drape.
- Raise a local anesthetic skin wheal just below the interlaminar space, about 0.5 cm from the midline toward the symptomatic side.
- Advance the Tuohy needle, angling slightly toward the midline until resistance of the ligamentum flavum is encountered, keeping the trajectory just lateral to the midline to avoid contacting the spinous process. Repeat imaging periodically to ensure that the needle is approaching the space, not the lamina or spinous process (see *Fig. 3.1.9*). Advance the needle through the ligamentum flavum using a loss of resistance technique with air or saline. Once loss of resistance is achieved, obtain a lateral view to ensure the needle is barely into the bony spinal canal.

- Attach a low volume extension set to the needle, aspirate to ensure there is no blood return, and inject 0.5–1 ml of non-ionic contrast medium during live fluoroscopy. Dye should be seen spreading within the bony canal (see *Fig. 3.1.10*). Prior to injecting local anesthetic or steroid, obtain an AP view to reconfirm epidural spread.

- Aspirate again, then inject local anesthetic (1–2 ml) and 50 mg triamcinolone diacetate or equivalent.
- Loss of resistance is occasionally encountered with the needle superficial to the epidural space. Dye will be seen dorsal to the epidural space on the lateral view, and spread lateral to the spinal canal will be seen on the AP view. The needle can then be advanced through the ligamentum flavum, again using loss of resistance, followed by dye confirmation.

Confirmation of a successful block

- Relief of pain.
- Anesthesia in the distribution of the blocked nerves.
- For lumbar epidural steroid injection, improvement in straight-leg raising may be evident.

Tips

- Air may be used instead of NaCl to determine loss of resistance. If this technique is used it is advisable to avoid constant pressure on the plunger, as the air is compressible; instead it should be bounced intermittently with the thumb to test for resistance and loss of resistance.
- Advocates claim identification of CSF is easier with this technique.
- Advocates of the use of NaCl point out that absolute resistance to pressure identifies the ligamentum flavum, and that by applying constant pressure to the plunger one can identify loss of resistance earlier, thereby more easily avoiding the possibility of dural tap.
- An epidural catheter may be inserted through the needle and the needle removed, taking care not to withdraw the catheter when removing the needle. However, a test dose of lidocaine (lignocaine) 1% 4 ml with/without epinephrine (adrenaline) 1:200 000 is given after insertion, before any injection through the catheter is carried out.
- Ultrasound may guide the insertion of the needle as spinous proccesses are easily visible on ultrasound (optional) (*Fig. 3.1.11*).

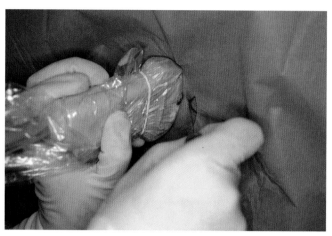

Fig. 3.1.11

- Injection of radio-opaque dye under direct fluoroscopy can confirm epidural placement.
- Insertion of a radio-opaque epidural catheter may be carried out also under fluoroscopy.

Potential problems

IMMEDIATE

- Failure to locate epidural space (sitting position may be successful).
- Intravascular injection (test dose important); addition of epinephrine (adrenaline) to test dose may help identification of intravascular injection.
- Intrathecal injection (test dose important).
- Hypotension due to sympathetic blockade (give i.v. fluid; consider ephedrine).
- Headache (possible dural puncture).
- Allergic reaction.

LATER

- Infection (epidural abscess; bacterial meningitis).
- Aseptic meningitis; usually a result of intrathecal injection (test dose important).
- Cushingoid symptoms; usually as a result of repeated steroid injections.

3.2 THORACIC EPIDURAL BLOCK

Anatomy

In the thoracic region, the spinous processes lie at an angle of 30–45° to the thoracic vertebral body (Fig. 3.2.1 a,b) thus making midline epidural injection a little more difficult, and sometimes necessitating a paramedian approach (Fig. 3.2.2 a–d).

Equipment

- 2 ml and 10 ml syringes
- 18 G, 20 G, and 25 G needles
- ECG, BP, and SpO$_2$ monitors
- 18 G epidural set
- Resuscitation equipment (*see Appendix 3*)
- Fluoroscopy or ultrasound (optional)

Drugs

- Lidocaine (lignocaine) 1%, 10 ml (or its equivalent)
- Corticosteroid if indicated, e.g. triamcinolone diacetate 50 mg (or its equivalent)
- Saline (NaCl) 10 ml
- Resuscitation drugs (*see Appendix 3*)

Position of patient

- Lateral, usually lying on the side of the radiculopathy.
- Shoulders and buttocks parallel to the edge of the bed, perpendicular to the floor, with spine flexed.

Needle puncture and technique

- Intravenous access is inserted.
- Monitors are attached.
- Resuscitation equipment and drugs are checked and made ready for use.
- The midline and an area 10 cm × 5 cm laterally is cleaned with antiseptic solution and a fenestrated drape is placed over the sterile area.
- Lidocaine (lignocaine) 1% 2 ml is drawn up into three 2 ml syringes.
- Lidocaine (lignocaine) 1% 2 ml, plus corticosteroid, e.g. triamcinolone diacetate 50 mg, is drawn up into the 10 ml syringe.
- NaCl 10 ml is drawn up into the 10 ml loss-of-resistance syringe.
- The spinous processes are palpated, and the level requiring injection is identified.
- This may be confirmed by fluoroscopy or ultrasound.

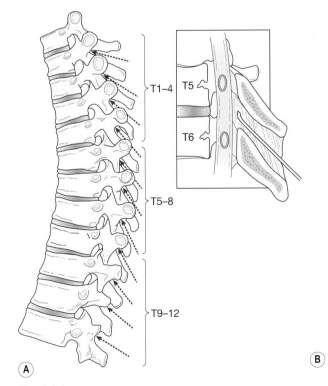

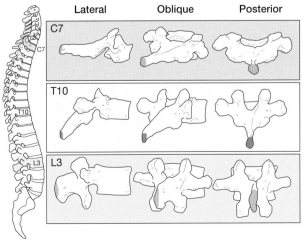

Fig. 3.2.1

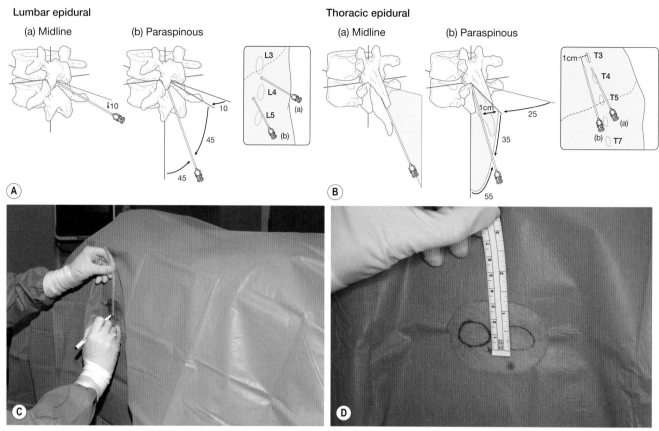

Lumbar epidural

(a) Midline   (b) Paraspinous

Thoracic epidural

(a) Midline   (b) Paraspinous

Fig. 3.2.2

Paramedian approach

FOR THE RIGHT-HANDED OPERATOR

With the left hand

- The fore- and middle fingers are placed each side of the interspace.
- These fingers are kept in place until the epidural needle is gripped by the interspinous ligament.

With the right hand

- The interspinous ligament is infiltrated with lidocaine (lignocaine) 1% 2 ml.
- **The insertion point of the epidural needle in the paravertebral approach lies 1 cm lateral to the midline, at the lower border of the spinous process** (*Fig. 3.2.3 a,b*). The epidural needle is inserted, bevel facing the side of radiculopathy, between the fore- and middle fingers of the left hand, perpendicular to the spine, parallel to the floor, until it is gripped by the interspinous ligament.
- **The direction of the needle is 130° cephalad and 15° medial to the midline.** Care must be taken as the ligamentum flavum is not as thick laterally, and may not be identified as easily. Therefore, it is usually easiest to first identify the lamina and **walk the needle off the**

lamina in a cephalad direction until the needle enters the ligamentum flavum. At that point the loss-of-resistance technique may be performed.

- The hub of the needle is gripped with the fore- and middle fingers of the left hand and this hand is steadied by leaning the wrist against the patient's back.
- The stylet is removed and the loss-of-resistance syringe is applied.
- The needle is slowly and carefully advanced until the osseous endpoint of the lamina is encountered.
- It is then walked off the lamina in the cephalad direction until it enters the ligamentum flavum.
- At the point at which the needle enters the ligamentum flavum, absolute resistance to injection is experienced.
- It is then carefully advanced further while constant pressure is applied to the plunger, the left hand aiding the advance, while at the same time applying a brake if required (*Fig. 3.2.4*, viewed from above).
- The needle is advanced very slowly until a sudden loss of resistance to the pressure on the plunger is experienced, the point at which the epidural space is entered.
- After negative aspiration for blood or cerebrospinal fluid, lidocaine (lignocaine) 1% 2 ml is injected.

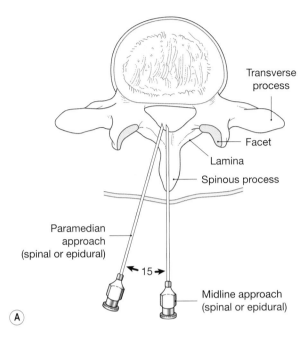

Transverse
process

Facet

Lamina

Spinous process

Paramedian
approach
(spinal or epidural)

←15→

Midline approach
(spinal or epidural)

(A)

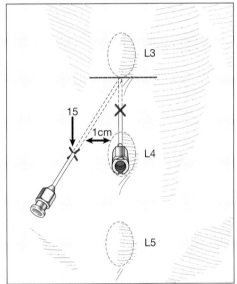

L3

15

1cm

L4

L5

(B)

Fig. 3.2.3

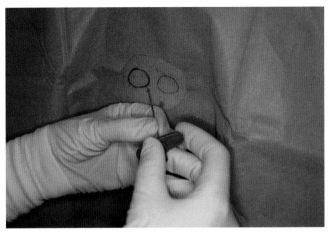

Fig. 3.2.4

- After 5 minutes the patient is questioned about changes in sensation or power, and any changes in heart rate or blood pressure are noted.
- If the injection is for diagnostic purposes only, the needle may be removed at this point.
- If therapeutic effect is required, lidocaine (lignocaine) 1% 2 ml plus corticosteroid, e.g. triamcinolone diacetate 50 mg, may be injected.
- The patient is allowed to lie in the lateral position, on the side of the pain.
- Monitors should be left attached and i.v. access should remain in situ for at least 30 minutes.

- The patient is advised to contact the hospital should anesthesia remain after several hours.

Confirmation of a successful block

- Relief of pain.
- Anesthesia in the distribution of blocked nerves.
- For lumbar epidural steroid injection, improvement in straight-leg raising may be evident.

Tips

- Air may be used instead of NaCl to determine loss of resistance. If this technique is used it is advisable to avoid constant pressure on the plunger, as the air is compressible; instead the plunger should be bounced intermittently with the thumb to test for resistance and loss of resistance.
- Advocates claim identification of CSF is easier with this technique.
- Advocates of the use of NaCl point out that absolute resistance to pressure identifies the ligamentum flavum, and that by applying constant pressure to the plunger one can identify loss of resistance more immediately, thereby avoiding the possibility of dural tap more easily.
- An epidural catheter may be inserted through the needle and the needle removed, taking care not to withdraw the catheter when removing the needle. However, a test dose of lidocaine (lignocaine) 1% 4 ml with epinephrine (adrenaline) 1:200 000 is given after insertion, before any injection through the catheter is carried out.
- Identification of the insertion point may be aided by ultrasound (*Fig. 3.2.5*).
- Injection of radio-opaque dye under direct fluoroscopy can confirm epidural placement.
- Insertion of a radio-opaque epidural catheter may be carried out also under fluoroscopy.

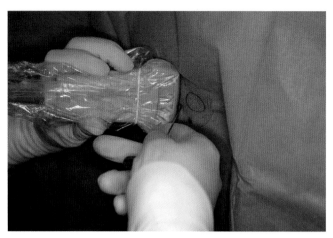

Fig. 3.2.5

Potential problems

IMMEDIATE
- Failure to locate epidural space (sitting position may be successful).

- Intravascular injection (test dose important); addition of epinephrine (adrenaline) to test dose may help identification of intravascular injection.
- Intrathecal injection (test dose important).
- Hypotension due to sympathetic blockade (give i.v. fluid, consider ephedrine).
- Headache (possible dural puncture).
- Allergic reaction.
- Spinal cord injury may occur if the epidural space is not recognized. Deep sedation should be avoided during needle insertion and drug injection.

LATER
- Infection (epidural abscess, bacterial meningitis).
- Aseptic meningitis, usually the result of intrathecal injection (test dose important).
- Cushingoid symptoms (usually as a result of repeated injections).
- Epidural hematoma. This complication should be suspected when sensory or motor function loss occurs minutes to hours after the procedure. Immediate diagnostic imaging (CT or MRI) is essential. Prompt surgical decompression may be required.

3.3 CERVICAL EPIDURAL BLOCK

Anatomy

In the cervical region, the spinous processes are almost perpendicular to the vertebral bodies, especially in the lower part. They also widen and become bifid. As a result, insertion of the needle is often easy. However, it must be remembered that the epidural space is relatively narrow in this area (2–4 mm), and that the spinal cord lies very close to it (Fig. 3.3.1 a,b). Most workers prefer to use the "hanging drop" technique when accessing the cervical epidural space, as there exists a significant negative pressure in the cervical region in the sitting position.

Equipment

- 2 ml, 5 ml, and 10 ml syringes
- 18 G, 20 G, and 25 G needles
- ECG, BP, and SpO$_2$ monitors
- 18 G epidural set
- Resuscitation equipment (*see Appendix 3*)
- Fluoroscopy or ultrasound (optional)

Drugs

- Lidocaine (lignocaine) 1%, 10 ml (or its equivalent)
- Corticosteroid if indicated, e.g. triamcinolone diacetate 50 mg (or its equivalent)
- Saline (NaCl) 10 ml
- Resuscitation drugs (*see Appendix 3*)

Position of patient

- Sitting.
- Head flexed forward.

Needle puncture and technique

- Intravenous access is inserted.
- Monitors are attached.
- Resuscitation equipment and drugs are checked and made ready for use.
- The midline and an area 10 cm × 5 cm laterally is cleaned with antiseptic solution and a fenestrated drape is placed over the sterile area.
- Lidocaine (lignocaine) 1% 2 ml is drawn up into two 2 ml syringes.
- Lidocaine (lignocaine) 1% 1 ml plus corticosteroid, e.g. triamcinolone diacetate 50 mg, is drawn up into a 5 ml syringe.
- NaCl 10 ml is drawn up into a 10 ml syringe.
- The patient is allowed to sit up straight for a moment, and the spinous process of T3, which lies opposite the

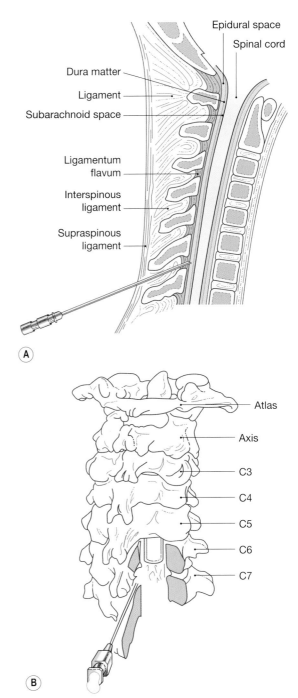

Fig. 3.3.1

root of the spine of the scapula, is identified and marked. The prominent spinous process of C7 (vertebra prominens) is identified (*Fig. 3.3.2*) and marked (*Fig. 3.3.3 a,b*). Ultrasound can be used to guide needle placement (*Fig. 3.3.3 c,d*). The interspace to be used for epidural injection is also marked.

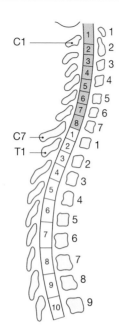

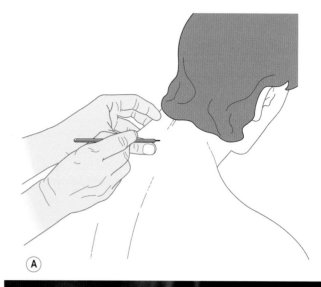

Fig. 3.3.2

FOR THE RIGHT-HANDED OPERATOR

With the left hand

- The fore- and middle fingers are placed each side of the interspace.
- These fingers are kept in place until the epidural needle is gripped by the interspinous ligament.

With the right hand

- The interspinous ligament is infiltrated with lidocaine (lignocaine) 1% 2 ml.
- **The epidural needle is inserted, bevel facing caudad, between the fore- and middle fingers of the left hand in a direction 60° cephalad, until it is gripped firmly by the interspinous ligament.**
- The hub of the needle is gripped with the fore- and middle fingers of the left hand and this hand is steadied by leaning the wrist against the patient's spine.
- The stylet is removed.
- The hub of the epidural needle is filled with saline (*Fig. 3.3.4*) such that a "hanging drop" appears (*Fig. 3.3.5*).

With both hands

- The wings of the epidural needle are gripped with each hand, steadying the hands by resting the wrists against the posterior thoracic wall (*Fig. 3.3.6*).
- The needle is slowly and carefully advanced with both hands.
- It is prudent periodically to confirm high resistance of the needle in the ligament by testing with an air-filled syringe, then replace the stylet to make sure there is no tissue blocking the needle before resuming the "hanging drop" technique.

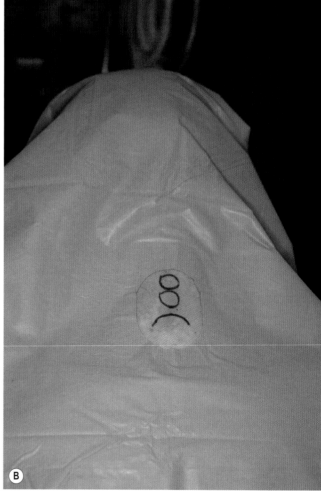

Fig. 3.3.3

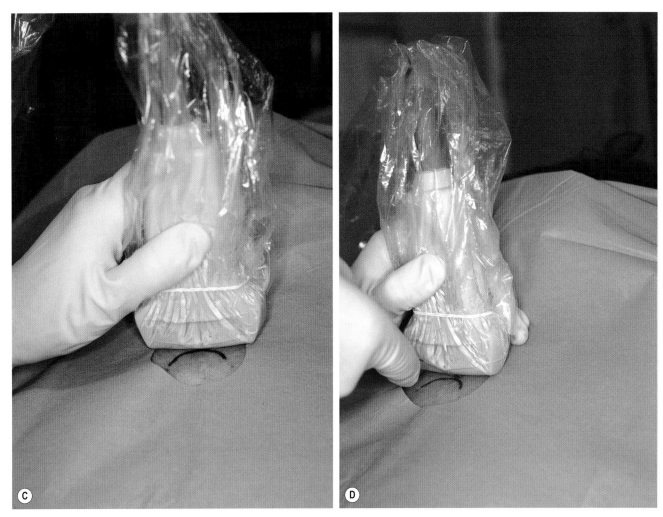

Fig. 3.3.3, cont'd

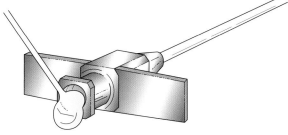

Fig. 3.3.4

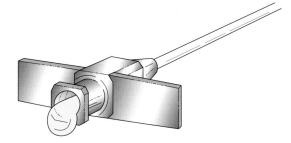

Fig. 3.3.5

- The "hanging drop" at the hub of the needle is watched closely, and the patient is asked periodically about the presence of paresthesia.
- At the point at which the epidural needle enters the epidural space, the drop should appear to be sucked into the needle (*Figs 3.3.7, 3.3.8*).
- After negative aspiration for blood or CSF, lidocaine (lignocaine) 1% 2 ml is injected.
- After 1–2 minutes the patient is questioned about changes in sensation or power, and any changes in heart rate or blood pressure are noted.
- If the injection is for diagnostic purposes only, the needle may be removed at this point.
- If therapeutic effect is required, lidocaine (lignocaine) 1% 1 ml plus corticosteroid, e.g. triamcinolone diacetate 50 mg, may be injected.
- The patient is allowed to lie in the lateral position, on the side of the pain.
- Monitors should be left attached and i.v. access kept in situ for at least 30 minutes.

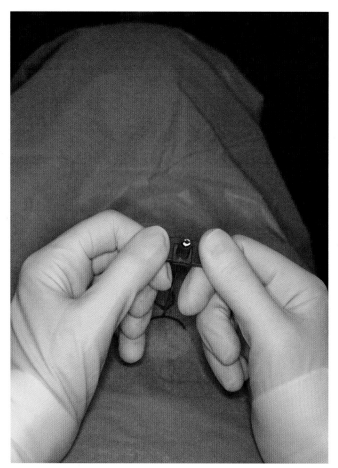

Fig. 3.3.6

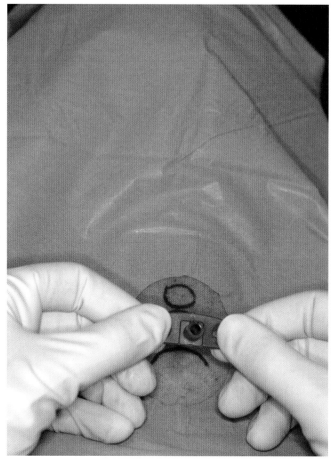

Fig. 3.3.8

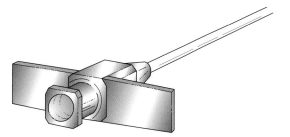

Fig. 3.3.7

- Ultrasound may aid in identifying the interspinous space as spinous processes are easily visible.

FLUOROSCOPIC GUIDED CERVICAL EPIDURAL INJECTION

- Check MRI to ensure that the spinal cord is not displaced posteriorly. If the posterior epidural space is compromised or the spinal cord is shifted posteriorly, it is safer to enter the upper thoracic epidural space and advance a radio-opaque catheter to the low cervical level.
- Position patient prone, with pillow under shoulders, neck flexed, arms at sides, shoulders as far downward as possible.

- Identify targeted interlaminar space (T1–2, C7–T1, or C6–7) in direct AP fluoroscopic view. Adjust angle upward or downward slightly to maximize view of interlaminar space.
- Mark skin over lower border of T1–2, C7–T1 (preferred) or C6–7 interlaminar space just lateral to the midline. Do not perform epidural injection above C6–7 because of absence of midline epidural fat at higher levels.
- Prepare skin with antiseptic and sterile drape.
- Provide only minimal sedation or no sedation. Instruct patient to report any pain or paresthesia during the procedure.
- Infiltrate skin and subcutaneous tissue with lidocaine (lignocaine) 1%.
- Advance the Tuohy needle through the insertion point into the interspinous ligament and check the fluoroscopy image to ensure the needle tip is directed toward the midline (*Fig. 3.3.9*).
- Begin to advance through the ligament using loss of resistance with air or saline. Check lateral view if possible (may be obscured by the shoulders). Proceed with needle advancement. When loss of resistance

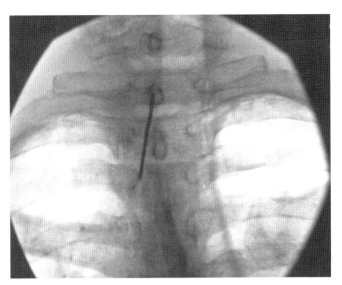

Fig. 3.3.9

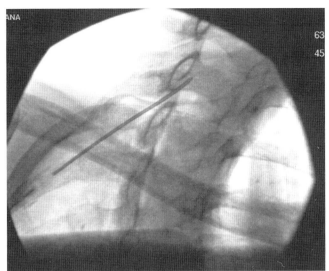

Fig. 3.3.10

occurs, recheck the lateral view. If unable to visualize the spinal canal, obtain slightly oblique view (*Fig. 3.3.10*).

- Attach a low volume extension set to the needle and inject a small volume (1 ml or less) of non-ionic contrast medium under live fluoroscopy, preferably in lateral view (AP or oblique view is used if this is not possible) (*Fig. 3.3.11*), then observe the AP view to confirm epidural dye spread.
- Aspirate to ensure there is no blood return, then inject 1–2 ml lidocaine (lignocaine) 1% followed by 25–50 mg triamcinolone diacetate or equivalent.

Confirmation of a successful block
- Relief of pain.

Tips
- Loss-of-resistance techniques may also be used to access the cervical epidural space.
- The steroid may be given soon after the test dose, as hypotension may be a problem if the patient remains in the sitting position.

Potential problems

IMMEDIATE
- Failure to locate epidural space (lateral position with loss of resistance technique may be successful).
- Pain on injection (caution: close proximity to spinal cord).
- Intrathecal injection (test dose important).
- Hypotension ± bradycardia due to sympathetic blockade (maximum 3 ml local anesthetic administered in this technique).
- Vasovagal syncope is common in young adult patients.

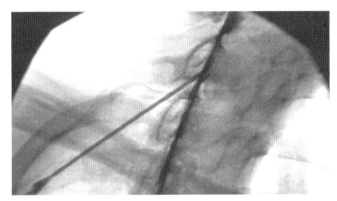

Fig. 3.3.11

- Intravascular injection; addition of epinephrine (adrenaline) 1:200 000 to the test dose may aid identification of intravascular injection.
- Headache (possible dural puncture).
- Allergic reaction.
- Spinal cord injury may occur if the epidural space is not recognized. Deep sedation should be avoided during needle insertion and drug injection.

LATER
- Infection (epidural abscess, bacterial meningitis).
- Aseptic meningitis, usually the result of intrathecal injection (test dose important).
- Cushingoid symptoms (usually as a result of repeated injections).
- Epidural hematoma. This complication should be suspected when sensory or motor function loss occurs minutes to hours after the procedure. Immediate diagnostic imaging (CT or MRI) is essential. Prompt surgical decompression may be required.

3.4 CAUDAL EPIDURAL BLOCK

Anatomy

Injection of anesthetic through the sacral hiatus allows access to the sacral epidural space or caudal anesthesia. The sacrum is roughly triangular in shape and is made up of five fused sacral vertebrae (Fig. 3.4.1). Its dorsal aspect is convex and there is a midline sacral canal that allows passage of the sacral nerves through four pairs of foramen, anteriorly and posteriorly. At the caudal end lies the coccyx, and at the cephalad end lies the fifth lumbar vertebra. The posterior wall of S5, and sometimes S4, is unfused. The thick fibrous sacro-coccygeal membrane or sacral hiatus covers the defect. This may be variable in size as the posterior wall of other sacral vertebrae may also be unfused. Penetration of this membrane allows access to the sacral epidural space.

Equipment

- 2 ml, 5 ml, and 20 ml syringes
- 18 G, 20 G, and 25 G needles
- 22 G, 3–5 cm short-bevel needle, with stylet
- ECG, BP, and SpO_2 monitors
- Resuscitation equipment (*see Appendix 3*)
- Fluoroscopy or ultrasound (optional)

Drugs

- Lidocaine (lignocaine) 1%, 10 ml (or its equivalent)
- Corticosteroid if indicated, e.g. triamcinolone diacetate 50 mg (or its equivalent)
- Saline (NaCl) 10 ml
- Resuscitation drugs (*see Appendix 3*)

Position of patient

- Prone.
- Pillow under abdomen and/or operating table broken to allow flexion of the lumbo-sacral spine.
- Lower limbs abducted 15°, toes rotated to point towards the opposite foot (*Fig. 3.4.2*).

Needle puncture and technique (adult)

- Intravenous access is inserted.
- Monitors are attached.
- Resuscitation equipment and drugs are checked and made ready for use.
- The midline and an area 10 cm × 5 cm laterally is cleaned with antiseptic solution and a fenestrated drape is placed over the sterile area.

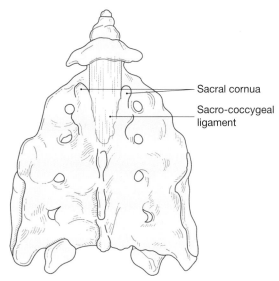

Sacral cornua

Sacro-coccygeal ligament

Fig. 3.4.1

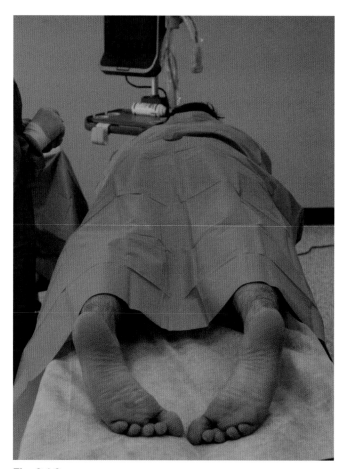

Fig. 3.4.2

- Lidocaine (lignocaine) 1% 2 ml is drawn up into three 2 ml syringes.
- Lidocaine (lignocaine) 1% 15 ml plus corticosteroid, e.g. triamcinolone diacetate 50 mg, is drawn up into the 20 ml syringe.
- NaCl 10 ml is drawn up into the 10 ml syringe.

FOR THE RIGHT-HANDED OPERATOR

With the left hand
- The posterior superior iliac spines are identified.
- The sacral cornua (the unfused spinous processes of S5) are also identified and marked.
- Between the cornua lies the base of the sacral hiatus, a roughly triangular fibroelastic structure.
- The index and middle fingers of the left hand are placed on each of the sacral cornua (*Fig. 3.4.3*).
- **The insertion point lies between these two fingers.**

With the right hand
- The insertion point is infiltrated with lidocaine (lignocaine) 1% 2 ml.
- The 22 G short-bevel needle with stylet is inserted at an angle of 45° to the skin (*Fig. 3.4.4. a,b*). Ultrasound can be used to guide needle placement (*Fig. 3.4.4c*).
- As the needle passes through the fibroelastic sacral hiatus, a "pop" may be experienced, although this is not always evident in adults, and bone may be contacted.
- After passing through the sacral hiatus, the needle is withdrawn a little, and redirected to an angle to the skin of 15–20° (*Fig. 3.4.5*). This should allow further advancement of 1–2 cm, as the needle enters the long axis of the caudal epidural space.
- After negative aspiration, lidocaine (lignocaine) 1% 2 ml is injected.

- After 5 minutes the patient is questioned about changes in sensation or power of the lower limbs, and any changes in heart rate or blood pressure are noted.
- Then lidocaine (lignocaine) 1% 5–15 ml plus corticosteroid, e.g. triamcinolone diacetate 50 mg, may be injected in order to promote spread to upper sacral and lower lumbar segments (a volume of at least 10 ml should be used if the symptoms are at the level of S1 nerve root or higher) (*Fig. 3.4.6*). The needle is then

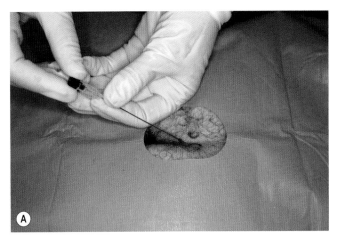

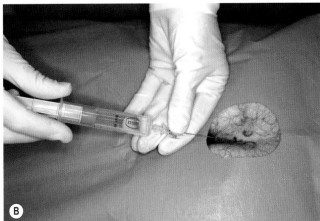

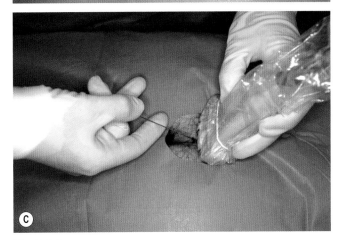

Fig. 3.4.4

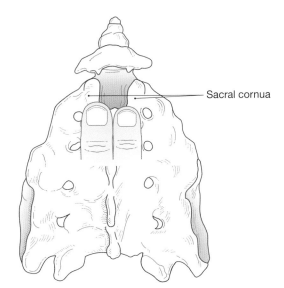

Sacral cornua

Fig. 3.4.3

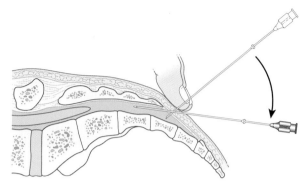

Fig. 3.4.5

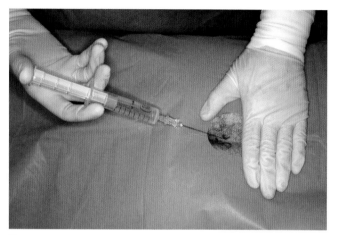

Fig. 3.4.6

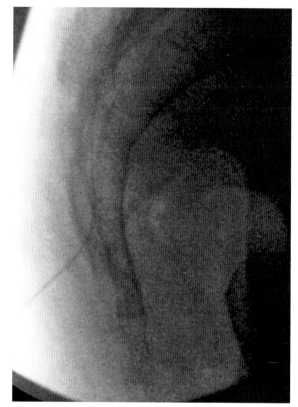

Fig. 3.4.7

removed while clearing it with lidocaine (lignocaine) 1% 2 ml.

- Monitors should be left attached and i.v. access kept in situ for at least 30 minutes.
- It is prudent to warn the patient about possible loss of sensation and or power of one or both lower limbs.

FLUOROSCOPIC GUIDED CAUDAL EPIDURAL INJECTION

- This approach may be used for treating L5 or S1 radiculopathy. It is a reasonable alternative to the interlaminar approach when surgery has disrupted the posterior spinal anatomy.
- Position the patient prone.
- Locate the sacral hiatus using the sacral cornua as landmarks.
- Prepare skin with antiseptic and sterile drape.
- Place the tip of a sterile blunt instrument over the sacral hiatus and obtain a lateral fluoroscopic view of the sacrum.
- Raise a skin wheal with 1% lidocaine (lignocaine) just below the sacral hiatus and infiltrate with lidocaine down to the sacral hiatus with a small gauge needle.

- Advance a Tuohy needle at a 45° angle to the skin through the sacral hiatus, checking a lateral fluoroscopic view to make sure the needle has entered the spinal canal. Lower the needle angle and advance the needle slightly. Recheck lateral fluoroscopy to ensure the needle is in the spinal canal.
- Aspirate to rule out intravascular placement and inject 0.5–1 ml contrast medium under live fluoroscopy. Check a lateral and AP image to ensure epidural spread.
- If no epidural catheter is used, inject a mixture of local anesthetic and steroid. Inject 10 ml 0.5% lidocaine plus 50 mg triamcinolone diacetate. This volume should be sufficient to reach the L5 or S1 nerve roots.
- Alternatively, a radio-opaque catheter can be inserted through the needle and advanced to the desired level. Check the catheter position in both AP and lateral views (*Fig. 3.4.7*). Attach the injection hub to the catheter and inject 0.5–1 ml contrast medium under live fluoroscopy, rechecking dye spread in both AP and lateral views (*Fig. 3.4.8*). Inject 1–2 ml 1% lidocaine plus 50 mg triamcinolone diacetate or equivalent.

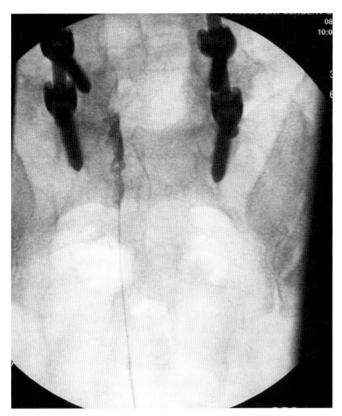

Fig. 3.4.8

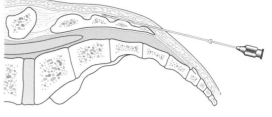

Fig. 3.4.9

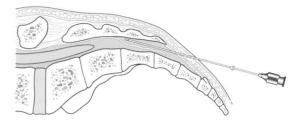

Fig. 3.4.10

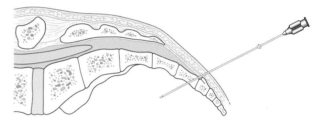

Fig. 3.4.11

Confirmation of a successful block

- Relief of pain.
- Anesthesia or diminished sensation in distribution of blocked nerves.
- Improvement in straight-leg raising (although for sacral nerve root-related pain, this may not have been positive prior to caudal blockade).

Tips

- After location of the caudal epidural space, the left hand may be placed over the sacral hiatus while 10 ml saline is rapidly injected (*Fig. 3.4.6*). Misplacement of the needle in the subcutaneous tissue (*Fig. 3.4.9*) should be evident if the injection is appreciated by the palpating left hand.
- Subperiosteal injection in the awake patient will cause pain (*Fig. 3.4.10*). The needle angle is important as the tip may come to lie anterior to the sacrum (*Fig. 3.4.11*).
- Anatomic variations exist in many patients, making access to the caudal epidural space difficult or impossible. Fluoroscopy using lateral views is useful to confirm the epidural needle position. Ultrasound may also be helpful in identifying the sacro-coccygeal membrane.

Potential problems

IMMEDIATE

- Failure to locate epidural space.
- Intravascular injection (test dose important); addition of epinephrine (adrenaline) to test dose may help identification of intravascular injection.
- Intrathecal injection, rare but possible (test dose important).
- Hypotension due to sympathetic blockade (give i.v. fluid, consider ephedrine).
- Transient exacerbation of radiculopathic pain (caution patient).
- Headache (possible dural puncture, rare).
- Allergic reaction.

LATER

- Infection (epidural abscess, bacterial meningitis).
- Aseptic meningitis, usually the result of intrathecal injection (test dose important).
- Cushingoid symptoms (usually as a result of repeated injections).
- Infection (epidural abscess).
- Epidural hematoma.

3.5 LONG-TERM EPIDURAL CATHETER INSERTION

Anatomy

As described for lumbar epidural block in Section 3.1.

Equipment

- 2 ml and 10 ml syringes
- 18 G, 20 G, and 25 G needles
- ECG, BP, and SpO$_2$ monitors
- 18 G epidural set
- Epidural catheter passer
- A surgical pack, including small scalpel and suture set
- Resuscitation equipment (*see Appendix 3*)
- Fluoroscopy or ultrasound (optional)

Drugs

- Lidocaine (lignocaine) 1% (preservative free) 20 ml (or its equivalent)
- Lidocaine (lignocaine) 1% (preservative free) 4 ml plus epinephrine (adrenaline) 1:200 000
- Saline (NaCl) 10 ml

Position of patient

- Lateral, lying on side of radiculopathy (*Fig. 3.5.1*).
- Shoulders and buttocks parallel to the edge of the bed, perpendicular to the floor, with spine flexed.

Needle puncture and technique

- Intravenous access is inserted.
- Monitors are attached.
- Resuscitation equipment and drugs are checked and made ready for use.
- The midline and an area 10 cm × 5 cm laterally is cleaned with antiseptic solution and a fenestrated drape is placed over the sterile area.
- Lidocaine (lignocaine) 1%, 2 ml is drawn up into three 2 ml syringes.
- Lidocaine (lignocaine) 1% 10 ml is drawn up into one 10 ml syringe.

- NaCl 10 ml is drawn up into the 10 ml loss-of-resistance syringe.
- An epidural catheter is inserted through the needle as previously described, 5–6 cm into epidural space (see Section 3.1).
- The needle is withdrawn 1–1.5 cm, but *is not removed*.
- After negative aspiration, a test dose of lidocaine (lignocaine) 1% 4 ml, with epinephrine (adrenaline) 1:200 000, is given. After 5 minutes the patient is questioned about changes in sensation or power, and any changes in heart rate or blood pressure are noted.
- After a negative reaction lidocaine (lignocaine) 1% 10 ml is injected slowly over 10 minutes. Assessment of the level of blockade is carried out after a further 15 minutes.
- Subcutaneous infiltration around the epidural needle with lidocaine (lignocaine) 1% is carried out. Note: a small incision is made to include the epidural needle (*Fig. 3.5.2*).
- A purse string suture is placed around the epidural needle, *but is not tied* (*Fig. 3.5.3*).
- Another small incision in the lateral abdominal wall is made after subcutaneous infiltration with lidocaine (lignocaine) 1% (*Fig. 3.5.4*). A catheter passer is tunneled through the subcutaneous tissue between the two incision sites.
- A catheter is manually bent to a curve and tunneled through the subcutaneous tissue between the two incision sites in the direction from the abdominal site to the epidural needle site (*Fig. 3.5.5*).
- The epidural needle is carefully removed (*Figs 3.5.6, 3.5.7*).
- The catheter is secured to subcutaneous tissue in the midline by tightening the purse string suture (*Fig. 3.5.8*).
- The catheter is further secured using an angle piece and then threaded in a lateral direction through the catheter

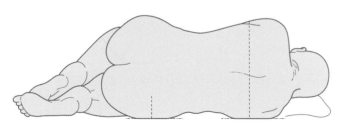

Fig. 3.5.1

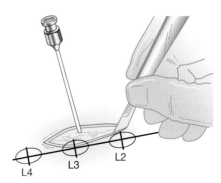

Fig. 3.5.2

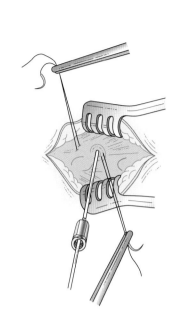

Fig. 3.5.3

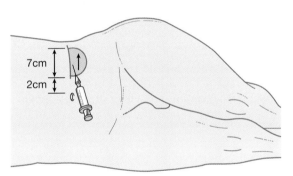

7cm

2cm

Fig. 3.5.4

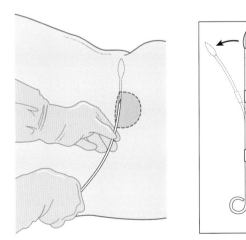

Fig. 3.5.5

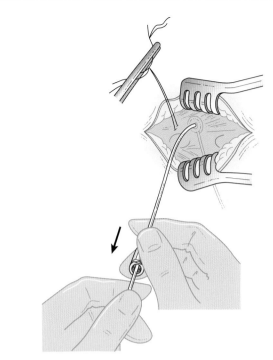

Fig. 3.5.6

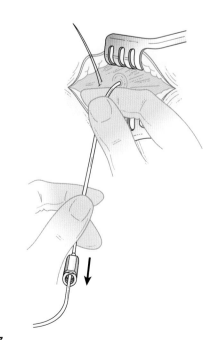

Fig. 3.5.7

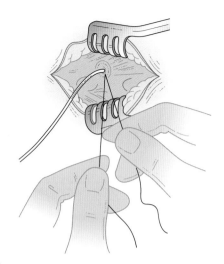

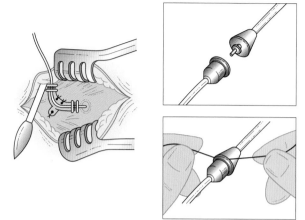

Fig. 3.5.8

Fig. 3.5.9

passer from the needle site to the abdominal wall site and connections are secured (*Fig. 3.5.9*).

- A pump may be placed in the abdominal wall site and the skin incisions closed.

Confirmation of a successful block

- Relief of pain.
- Anesthesia or diminished sensation in the distribution of affected nerves.

Tips

- Injection of radio-opaque dye under direct fluoroscopy can confirm epidural placement.

- Insertion of a radio-opaque epidural catheter may be carried out also under fluoroscopy.
- Ultrasound may aid insertion

Potential problems

- As described for lumbar epidural block in Section 3.1.
- However, in view of the long-term nature of epidural catheter implantation, any symptoms of infection should be immediately investigated and treated.
- Epidural catheters should not be inserted or removed during anticoagulation. Coagulation and platelet function should be normalized before catheter removal.

SOMATIC NERVE BLOCKADE

4

Mechanical nerve root compression was originally thought to be the cause of pain in discogenic radiculopathy. However, it has been found that many asymptomatic patients demonstrate substantial disc protrusion on magnetic resonance (MR) imaging, myelography and subsequent autopsy examination. In addition, surgical decompression does not result in uniform success in the relief of such pain. Following a period of mechanical nerve-root compression it is likely that an acute inflammatory process ensues, resulting in intraneural accumulation of serum proteins and fluid, raised intraneural pressure, ischemia and axonal degeneration. Degenerating glycoprotein material from the nucleus pulposis may also contribute to the inflammatory process.

There are many situations in which injection of spinal nerve roots with local anesthetic may be helpful in the diagnosis of radicular pain. These include those where investigations including electromyography, computer tomography (CT) or MR imaging are not consistent with the clinical findings, where there are multiple levels of pathology, and after spinal surgery with subsequent scarring in the area of the surgery. In addition, the contribution of the somatic nerve root may be elucidated in pain of uncertain origin, e.g. chest pain or abdominal pain, by specific nerve root local anesthetic injection.

It may be used therefore to determine the level of surgery, if indicated, and the addition of steroid may produce longer-lasting pain relief.

4.1 INTERCOSTAL NERVE BLOCK

Anatomy

The intercostal nerve is made up of several types of nerves: sympathetic white and grey rami communicantes, cutaneous and motor fibers supplied by dorsal rami, sensory fibers to the chest wall, anterior and posterior, via the lateral cutaneous branch, and further sensory fibers to the anterior chest wall via the anterior cutaneous branch. The lateral cutaneous branch exits just distal to the angle of the rib. Just below the inferior edge of the rib, in the intercostal groove, lie the intercostal nerve, artery and vein, the latter lying superior to the nerve. The optimal site to block the intercostal nerve is the most posterior point at which the rib is palpable, usually the angle of the rib (Fig. 4.1.1 a,b).

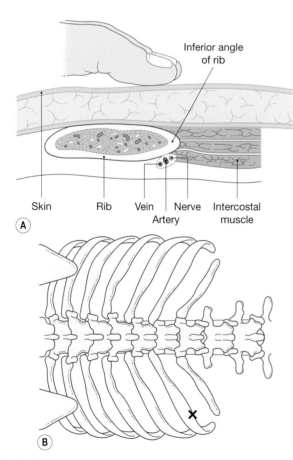

Fig. 4.1.1

Equipment

- 2 ml and 5 ml syringes
- 30 G needle
- 22 G 3–4 cm short-bevel needle
- Extension set (optional)
- ECG, BP, and SpO_2 monitors
- Resuscitation equipment (see Appendix 3)
- Ultrasound (optional)

Drugs

- Lidocaine (lignocaine) 1% 2 ml for skin infiltration
- Lidocaine (lignocaine) 1% 5 ml (or its equivalent)
- Corticosteroid if indicated, e.g. triamcinolone diacetate 50 mg (or its equivalent)
- Resuscitation drugs (see Appendix 3)

Position of patient

- Prone (this allows best access, although a lateral or supine position may also be used).
- Pillow under mid-abdomen to widen the intercostal spaces.
- Arms hanging over sides of table to rotate the scapulae laterally.

Needle puncture and technique

- Intravenous access is inserted.
- Monitors are attached.
- Resuscitation equipment and drugs are checked and made ready for use.
- Sedation may be administered if multiple blocks are being performed.
- The midline and an area 10 cm × 10 cm laterally is cleaned with antiseptic solution and a fenestrated drape is placed over the sterile area.
- The midline is palpated and marked.
- **The inferior edge of the rib is palpated and marked at the most posterior point at which the rib is palpable; this is the insertion point** (Fig. 4.1.2). If multiple blocks are planned these marks will form a line that becomes more medial towards the cephalad end as the scapulae are avoided laterally (Fig. 4.1.2).

FOR THE RIGHT-HANDED OPERATOR

With the left hand

- The inferior edge of the rib is palpated with the fore- and middle fingers (Fig. 4.1.3).

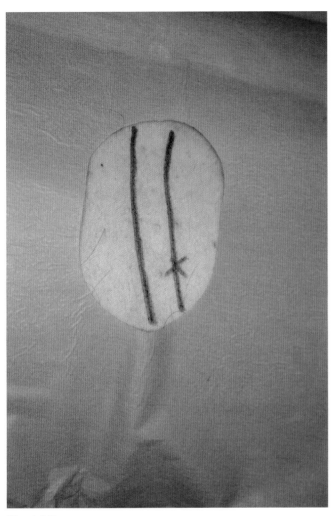

Fig. 4.1.2

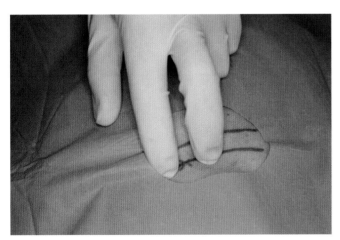

Fig. 4.1.3

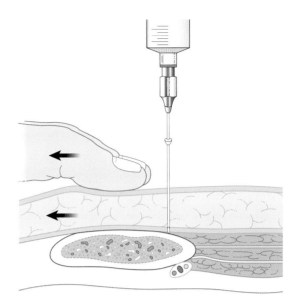

Fig. 4.1.4

- The skin is drawn up over the rib itself.
- The fingers of the left hand will grip the needle-hub for controlled advancement of the needle once contact with the rib is made during injection.

With the right hand
- The insertion point is infiltrated with lidocaine (lignocaine) 1% using a 2 ml syringe and a 30 G needle.
- The 22 G short-bevel needle with syringe attached is inserted between fore- and middle finger of the left hand in a direction 15–20° cephalad, until it makes contact with the rib (*Figs 4.1.4, 4.1.5*).
- The needle-hub is gripped with the fingers of the left hand and this hand is steadied by leaning the wrist against the patient's posterior chest wall.
- With the right and left hands acting as one unit, the needle is walked off the edge of the rib until it enters the intercostal space immediately below the rib (*Fig 4.1.6*). Alternatively, a catheter may be inserted between the needle and syringe and injection may then be carried out by a second operator, while the first maintains the needle steady in the correct position (*Fig. 4.1.7*).
- It is then advanced 2 mm.
- After negative aspiration, 3–4 ml of local anesthetic, plus corticosteroid if indicated, is injected and the needle is withdrawn.
- Monitors are left attached and i.v. access left in situ for at least 30 minutes.
- Chest X-ray is performed if pneumothorax is suspected.

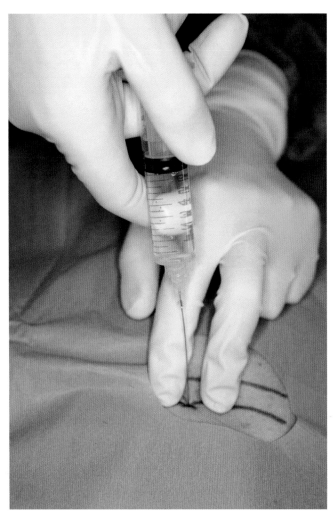

Fig. 4.1.5

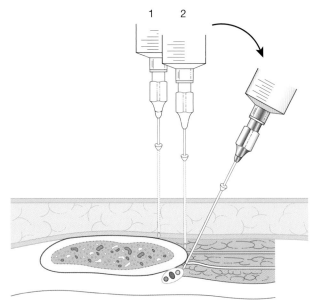

Fig. 4.1.6

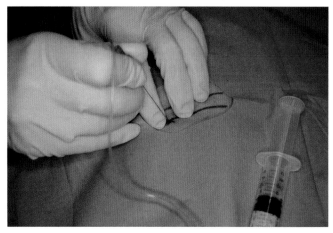

Fig. 4.1.7

Confirmation of a successful block

- Relief of pain.
- Anesthesia in the distribution of the blocked nerve.

Tips

- The approximate depth to the rib may be determined with the left fore- and middle fingers before insertion of the needle.
- Insertion of the needle > 2 mm deeper than the rib when intercostal space is reached is avoided. This will minimize the risk of pneumothorax, as the average distance from the rib to the pleura is 8 mm. If patient coughs on injection, pneumothorax is suspected.
- Neurolytic intercostal nerve block, e.g. with alcohol 50% 3 ml (made up by combining equal parts of alcohol 100% and lidocaine (lignocaine) 1% or its equivalent), or phenol 6%, may be carried out after local anesthetic block confirms accurate placement of the needle as described above. However, it is important to note that injection may result in subarachnoid spread of a neurolytic agent with resultant possible permanent spinal cord damage.
- Ultrasound may aid accurate placement of the needle (*Fig. 4.1.8*). Injection of non-ionic radio-constrast medium may also aid accurate placement of the needle in neurolytic block (*Fig. 4.1.9*).
- Placement of a catheter into the intercostal space can be achieved by threading 3 cm of catheter through an 18 G epidural needle after the intercostal neurovascular bundle has been identified as above.

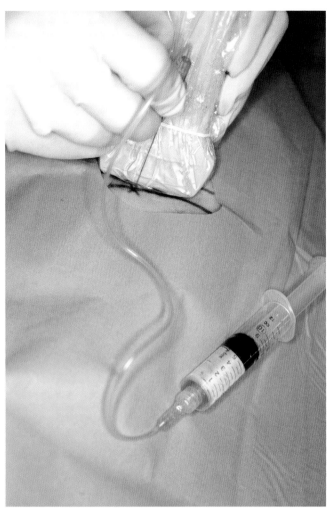

Fig. 4.1.8

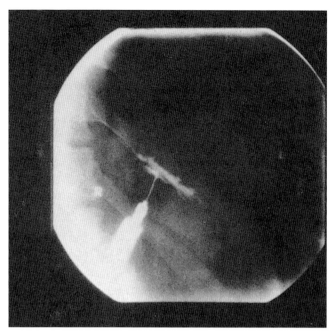

Fig. 4.1.9

Radiofrequency lesioning

- Radiofrequency lesioning of the intercostal nerve is simple and has a low level of side effects. The lesioning is carried out using the same method of placement of the needle as described for intercostal nerve block with local anesthetic.
- However, after placement of the needle and confirmation of accuracy by fluoroscopy (as described above), a trial of stimulation is carried out using 2 V at 50 Hz. If the needle has been placed accurately the patient should experience paresthesiae in the distribution of that intercostal nerve. A pulsed radiofrequency lesion may then be produced at 40–45 °C for 5 minutes or 49–60 °C for 90 seconds.

Potential problems

- Injection within the nerve sheath can result in the spread of anesthetic to the subarachnoid space.
- Intercostal block in patients with severe respiratory problems should be avoided as there is risk of a pneumothorax. Careful observation of a small pneumothorax is usually all that is required but failure to re-expand the lung may require chest tube insertion.
- Because of the vascularity of the intercostal space, there may be rapid absorption of local anesthetic and systemic effects can occur quickly, especially with multiple blocks. However, peak plasma concentration of local anesthetic may occur 15–20 minutes after the block is performed, when systemic toxicity effects may develop. Addition of epinephrine (adrenaline) to the anesthetic solution may decrease the peak plasma concentration of local anesthetic.
- If aspiration of blood occurs, the needle should be removed, keeping the left fore- and middle fingers in place. The needle is cleared, reinserted to contact the rib again, and the block is continued as above.

- Care of the airway must be remembered if sedation is administered to a patient in the prone position.
- Complications of neurolytic intercostal nerve block include pneumothorax, infection (especially in the immunocompromised patient) as well as post-lesioning intercostal nerve neuritis. The frequency of the latter in radiofrequency lesioning increases as higher temperatures are used. Intercostal nerve neuritis usually responds to local injection of lidocaine (lignocaine) 1% 3 ml plus triamcinolone diacetate 20 mg to the lesion site.

4.2 INTERPLEURAL BLOCK

Anatomy

The parietal pleura lines the thoracic wall, the thoracic surface of the diaphragm and the lateral mediastinum. The visceral pleura completely covers the surface of the lung. Both the pleural layers become contiguous at the root of the lung. Between the two pleural layers lies the interpleural space (Fig. 4.2.1). Injection of local anesthetic into this space produces an interpleural block by topical contact with free nerve endings within the pleura, and by local diffusion to nerves in the vicinity of the injection site. These include the intercostal nerves, the sympathetic chain, and the inferior part of the brachial plexus. Local anesthetic solution may also track to the epidural and subarachnoid spaces producing blockade.

Equipment

- 2 ml and 10 ml syringes
- 18 G, 20 G, and 25 G needles
- ECG, BP, and SpO_2 monitors
- 18 G epidural set
- Well-lubricated 5 ml glass syringe
- Resuscitation equipment (see Appendix 3)

Drugs

- Lidocaine (lignocaine) 1% 10 ml
- Levobupivacaine 0.25%, 20 ml (or its equivalent)
- Saline (NaCl) 10 ml
- Resuscitation drugs (see Appendix 3)

Position of patient

- The technique described here relies on negative interpleural pressure to identify the interpleural space. Therefore the patient should be breathing spontaneously for this technique.
- Semi-prone.
- Side to be blocked uppermost, supported by a pillow (Fig. 4.2.2).
- The arm should be allowed to fall forwards in front of the body to rotate the scapula anterolaterally.

Needle puncture and technique

- Intravenous access is inserted.
- Monitors are attached.
- Resuscitation equipment and drugs are checked and made ready for use.
- The midline and an area 15 cm × 12 cm laterally is cleaned with antiseptic solution and a fenestrated drape is placed over the sterile area.
- Lidocaine (lignocaine) 2%, 2 ml is drawn up.
- Levobupivacaine 0.25% 20 ml is drawn up.
- Air is drawn up into a well-lubricated 5 ml syringe.
- The seventh and eighth ribs are palpated and marked.

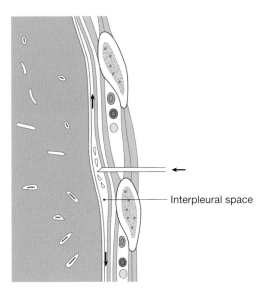

Interpleural space

Fig. 4.2.1

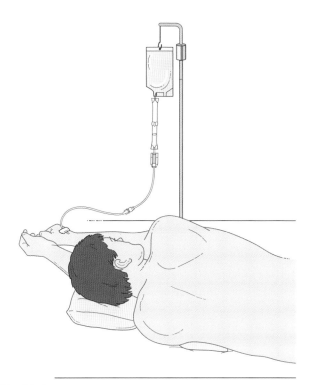

Fig. 4.2.2

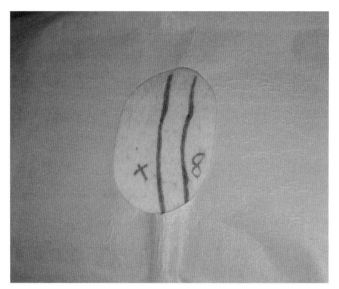

Fig. 4.2.3

- **A point approximately 10 cm from the midline, immediately superior to the eighth rib, is marked; this is the insertion point** (*Fig. 4.2.3*).

FOR THE RIGHT-HANDED OPERATOR

With the left hand
- The fore- and middle fingers are placed each side of the insertion point, palpating the superior aspect of the eighth rib.
- These fingers are kept in place until the epidural needle passes through the subcutaneous tissue.

With the right hand
- A skin wheal is raised at the insertion point.
- The epidural needle is inserted between the fore- and middle fingers of the left hand, taking care that the point of entry of the needle is as close as possible to the superior aspect of the eighth rib. This helps to avoid damage to the neurovascular bundle, which lies immediately inferior to the seventh rib.
- After passage through the subcutaneous tissue, the hub of the needle is gripped with the fore- and middle fingers of the left hand and this hand is steadied by leaning the wrist against the patient's posterior chest wall.
- The stylet is removed and the well-lubricated glass syringe containing 3 ml air is applied (*Fig. 4.2.4*).
- The needle is slowly and carefully advanced, with no pressure applied to the plunger, the left hand aiding the advance, while at the same time applying a brake if required.
- Resistance from the tissues prevents the plunger from advancing.
- At the point at which the needle enters the interpleural space a definite click is experienced, negative pressure draws the air in and the barrel drops (*Fig. 4.2.5*).

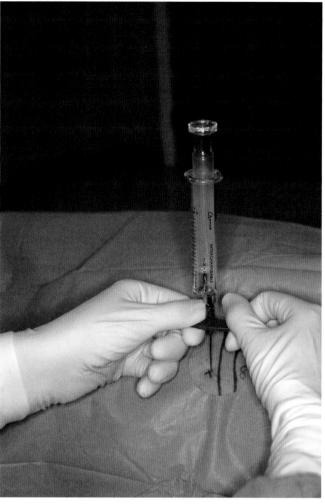

Fig. 4.2.4

- Taking care not to allow air entry into the interpleural cavity, a catheter is inserted approximately 10 cm into the interpleural space (*Fig. 4.2.6*). **Once the catheter is in position it is best to place the patient supine, tilted slightly, with the side to be blocked upwards** (*Fig. 4.2.7 a,b*). **(If blockade of the upper thoracic segments is required the patient is tilted head-down).**
- After negative aspiration and a test dose, 10–15 ml levobupivacaine 0.25% (or its equivalent) in divided doses of 5 ml is injected.
- Infusion of local anesthetic may be set up for continuous analgesia.
- Monitors should be left attached and i.v. access left in situ while the catheter is in place.
- Chest radiograph may be performed to rule out pneumothorax.

Confirmation of a successful block

- Relief of pain.
- Anesthesia in the distribution of the blocked nerves.

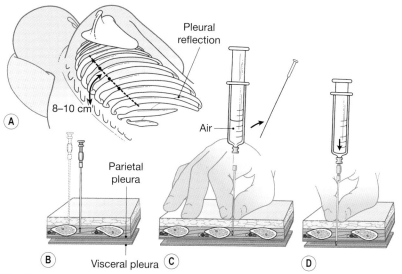

Pleural
reflection

8–10 cm

Air

Parietal
pleura

Visceral pleura

Fig. 4.2.5

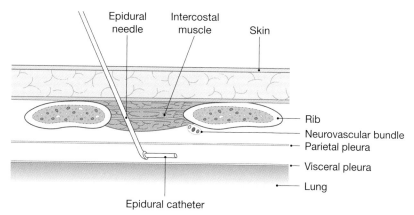

Epidural
needle

Intercostal
muscle

Skin

Rib

Neurovascular bundle

Parietal pleura

Visceral pleura

Lung

Epidural catheter

Fig. 4.2.6

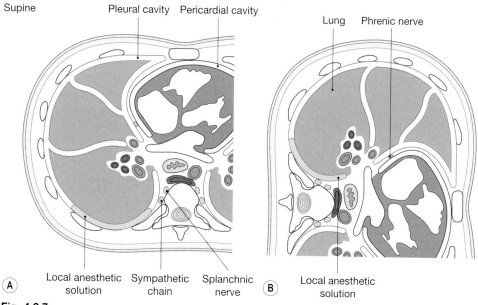

Supine

Pleural cavity   Pericardial cavity

Lung   Phrenic nerve

Local anesthetic
solution

Sympathetic
chain

Splanchnic
nerve

Local anesthetic
solution

Fig. 4.2.7

Tips

- As an alternative technique, the barrel of the syringe may be removed and the open syringe filled with NaCl or local anesthetic and advanced until the fluid level begins to fall as the solution is sucked into the interpleural space (*Fig. 4.2.8*).
- Also, a bag containing NaCl 500 ml may be attached to the epidural needle via a giving set, and drops observed on entry to the interpleural space (*Fig. 4.2.9*).
- Ultrasound may aid placement of the needle (*Fig. 4.2.10*).

Potential problems

- Pneumothorax.
- Unpredictable analgesia. The mechanism of action of interpleural block is still unproven and spread of the local anesthetic solution may be unpredictable. The duration of the block may be decreased when a thoracotomy drainage tube is present.

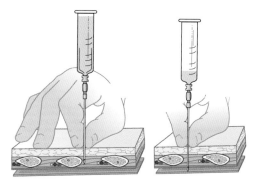

Fig. 4.2.8

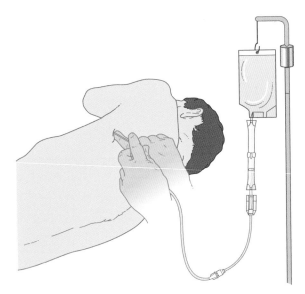

Fig. 4.2.9

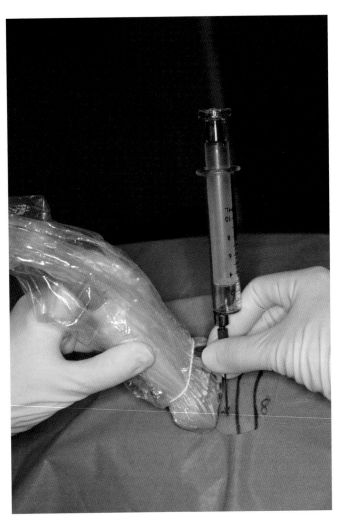

Fig. 4.2.10

4.3 LUMBAR NERVE ROOT BLOCK

Anatomy

The lumbar nerves are made up of sensory and motor fibers to the trunk and lower limbs, and sympathetic white and grey rami communicantes. Each lumbar nerve exits via the intervertebral foramen which lies just inferior to the caudad edge of the transverse process of the respective vertebral body, and passes anteriorly over the lateral aspect of the transverse process of the vertebral body below (Fig. 4.3.1). It then branches into posterior and anterior branches. The posterior branch supplies the paravertebral muscles and cutaneous fibers to the back. The anterior branch passes through the substance of the psoas muscle and branches further, communicating with the other anterior branches to form the lumbar plexus. As a result there is significant overlap of nerve supply. The fascial layers of the psoas muscle prevent spread of local anesthetic to the sympathetic lumbar chain. It may be helpful to consider blockade of a lumbar nerve root to be similar to intercostal nerve block except that the transverse process is present instead of a rib and the insertion site is therefore more medial.

Equipment

- 2 ml and 10 ml syringes
- 25 G needle

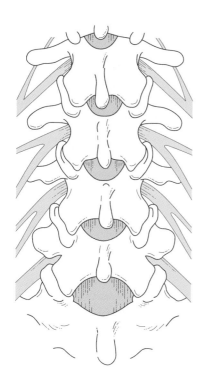

Fig. 4.3.1

- 22 G spinal needle, end-opening
- Radio-opaque contrast medium
- ECG, BP, and SpO$_2$ monitors
- Resuscitation equipment (*see Appendix 3*)
- Fluoroscopy or ultrasound

Drugs

- Lidocaine (lignocaine) 1% 10 ml (or its equivalent)
- Corticosteroid if indicated, e.g. triamcinolone diacetate 25 mg (or its equivalent)
- Resuscitation drugs

Position of patient

- Prone.
- Pillow under the anterior superior iliac spine to flatten the normal lumbar lordosis (*Fig. 4.3.2*).

Needle puncture and technique

- Intravenous access is inserted.
- Monitors are attached.
- Resuscitation equipment and drugs are checked and made ready for use.
- The lumbar midline and an area 10 cm × 5 cm laterally is cleaned with antiseptic solution and a fenestrated drape is placed over the sterile area.
- The iliac crests are palpated and the intercrestal line is identified. This corresponds with the inferior aspect of the spinous process of L4 or may lie in the L4–5 interspace (*Fig. 4.3.3 a*).
- The spinous processes are counted until the level to be blocked is identified and confirmed with fluoroscopy.
- The spinous processes of the vertebrae are marked (*Fig. 4.3.3 b*).
- **The insertion point of the needle lies 2–3 cm lateral to the cephalic end of the spinous process of the vertebra. The nerve corresponding to each vertebra emerges just below the transverse process of that vertebra at this site** (*see Appendix 6*).
- Therefore, with the aid of fluoroscopy, the insertion point is identified.
- A skin wheal is raised and the area is infiltrated with lidocaine (lignocaine) 1%.
- A spinal needle is introduced in a vertical direction to the skin, until the needle contacts bone at an approximate depth of 3–5 cm, the transverse process of that vertebra (*Fig. 4.3.4 a,b*).

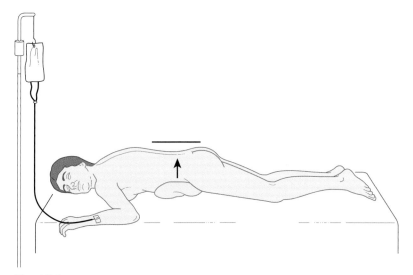

Fig. 4.3.2

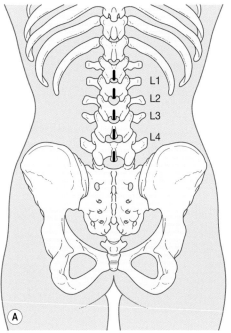

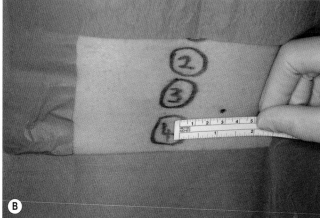

Fig. 4.3.3

- The needle is then walked off the transverse process in the caudad direction and advanced 1.5–2 cm, the site of the emerging nerve root (*Fig. 4.3.5*).
- It is useful to confirm the needle tip over the intervertebral foramen with fluoroscopy.
- Paresthesia in the distribution of the nerve may be experienced.
- After aspiration, non-ionic radio-opaque contrast medium 1 ml is injected.
- The correct placement is indicated by outlining the nerve root with non-ionic radio-opaque contrast medium,

visible on anteroposterior and lateral fluoroscopic views (*Fig. 4.3.6*).
- After further aspiration, lidocaine (lignocaine) 1% 0.5–1 ml is injected.
- After 5 minutes the patient is questioned about changes in pain, sensation and power of the lower limb.
- For diagnostic nerve root blockade, the needle may be removed when the level causing pain is identified.
- Ultrasound may also aid placement of the needle (*Fig. 4.3.7*).

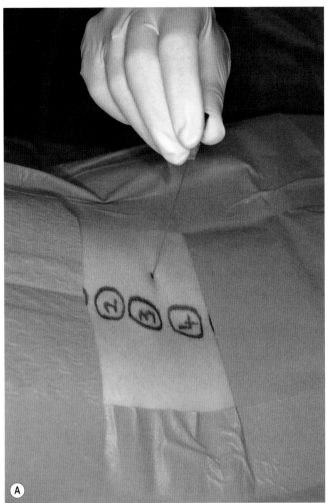

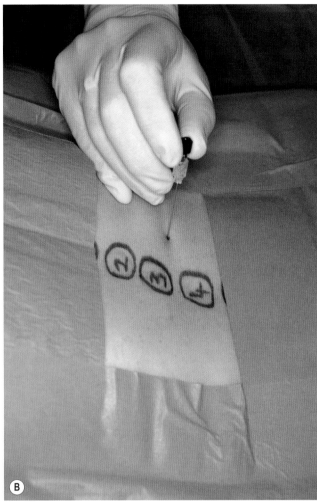

Fig. 4.3.4

Confirmation of a successful block

• Relief of pain and anesthesia in distribution of the blocked nerve.

Tips

• As in the case of thoracic nerve root block, it has also been recommended that the needle is angled 20° medially after entering the paravertebral space. However care must be taken, with the aid of fluoroscopy, not to inject local anesthetic solution into the nerve sheath allowing tracking of the solution centrally to produce intrathecal blockade.

Potential problems

• Intrathecal injection.
• Epidural blockade usually occurs with this block, but this is not a problem once low volumes are used.

However, even small volumes of epidural spread may confound the diagnostic value of the block.

• Sympathetic blockade is unlikely, but it may occur and cause hemodynamic changes.
• Intravascular injection. Injection of particulate steroids into a radicular artery can cause spinal cord infarction. Particulate steroids should never be injected near the foramen unless intravascular placement has been ruled out using live fluoroscopy contrast dye injection, preferably with digital subtraction technique.

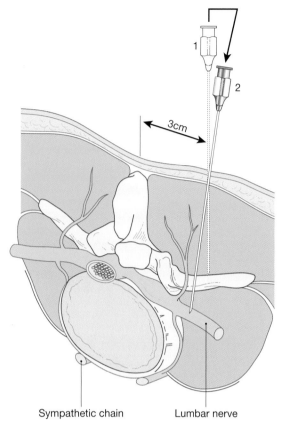

Fig. 4.3.5

Sympathetic chain   Lumbar nerve

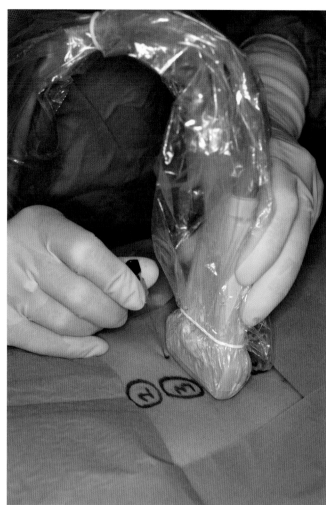

Fig. 4.3.7

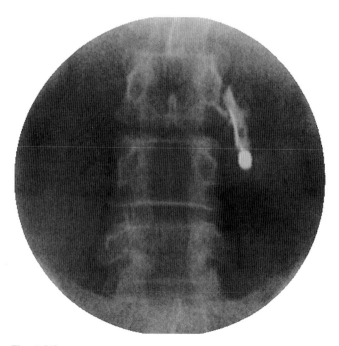

Fig. 4.3.6

4.4 THORACIC NERVE ROOT BLOCK

Anatomy

The anatomy relevant to thoracic paravertebral nerve root blockade is very similar to the anatomy relevant to lumbar paravertebral nerve root block, except that:

- ribs are present instead of the rudimentary ribs of the lumbar spine, the transverse processes;
- the lung and pleura are in close proximity to the injection site, therefore the risk of pneumothorax is significant;
- unlike the lumbar region, where the needle passes through the substance of the psoas muscle, the needle passes through connective tissue only in the thoracic region (*Fig. 4.4.1 a,b*);
- the fascial layers of the psoas muscle prevent spread to the sympathetic lumbar chain. However, such layers do not exist in the thoracic region, and paravertebral injection usually results in sympathetic blockade.

Equipment

- 2 ml and 10 ml syringes
- 25 G needle
- 22 G spinal needle, end-opening
- Radio-opaque contrast medium

- ECG, BP, and SpO_2 monitors
- Resuscitation equipment and drugs (*see Appendix 3*)
- Fluoroscopy or ultrasound

Drugs

- Lidocaine (lignocaine) 1% 10 ml (or its equivalent)
- Corticosteroid if indicated, e.g. triamcinolone diacetate 25 mg (or its equivalent)
- Resuscitation drugs (*see Appendix 3*)

Position of patient

- Prone (the block requires localization of the transverse process and can be performed in a lateral, sitting or prone position) (*Fig. 4.4.2*).

Needle puncture and technique

- Intravenous access is inserted.
- Monitors are attached.
- Resuscitation equipment and drugs are checked and made ready for use.
- The thoracic midline and an area 10 cm × 5 cm laterally is cleaned with antiseptic solution.

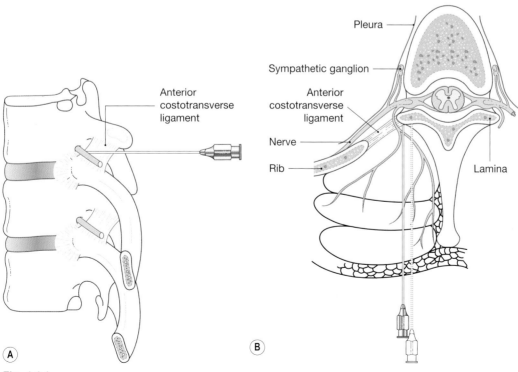

Anterior costotransverse ligament

Anterior costotransverse ligament

Pleura

Sympathetic ganglion

Nerve

Rib

Lamina

(A)

(B)

Fig. 4.4.1

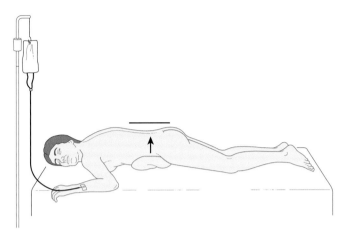

Fig. 4.4.2

- The inferior angle of the scapula is identified; this lies at the level of the spinous process of T7.
- The root of the spine of the scapula is identified; this lies at the level of the spinous process of T3.
- The spinous processes are counted until the level to be blocked is identified, and confirmed with fluoroscopy.
- The spinous processes of vertebrae are then marked.
- **The insertion point of the needle lies 1.5–3 cm lateral to the cephalic end of the spinous process of the vertebra, usually midway between the ribs** (*Fig. 4.4.3 a,b*).
- The nerve corresponding to each vertebra emerges just below the transverse process of that vertebra at this site.
- Therefore, with the aid of fluoroscopy, the insertion point is identified.
- A skin wheal is raised and the area is infiltrated with lidocaine (lignocaine) 1%.
- The transverse process is identified under fluoroscopy and the spinal needle is introduced in a direction perpendicular to the skin until the needle contacts bone.
- A slightly mesiad inclination avoids the pleura and increases the chances of placing the needle tip near the nerve root.
- Care must be taken to avoid the pleura by not advancing the needle any further than is necessary to locate the transverse process, approximately 3 cm. If the needle does not contact the transverse process by 3 cm, it should be withdrawn and re-advanced in a more caudad, and subsequently more cephalic, direction, again taking care not to advance beyond 3 cm.
- The needle is then walked off the caudad edge of the transverse process until it slips off the edge (*Fig. 4.4.4 a,b*). It is then advanced 1 cm, the site of the emerging nerve root at that level.
- It is useful to confirm the needle tip over the intervertebral foramen with fluoroscopy.
- Paresthesia in the distribution of the nerve may be experienced.

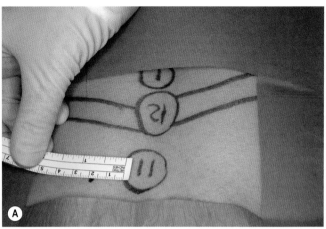

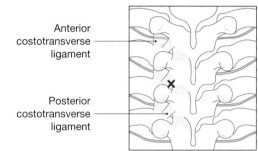

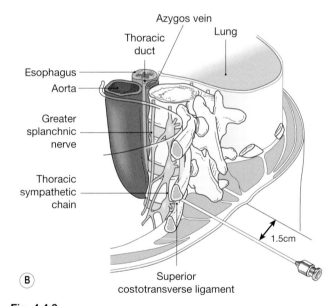

Fig. 4.4.3

- After aspiration, radio-opaque contrast medium 1 ml, is injected.
- The correct placement is indicated by outlining the nerve root with non-ionic radio-opaque contrast medium, visible on anteroposterior and lateral views (as in the description of lumbar somatic nerve injection in Section 4.3).
- Ultrasound may aid placement of needle.

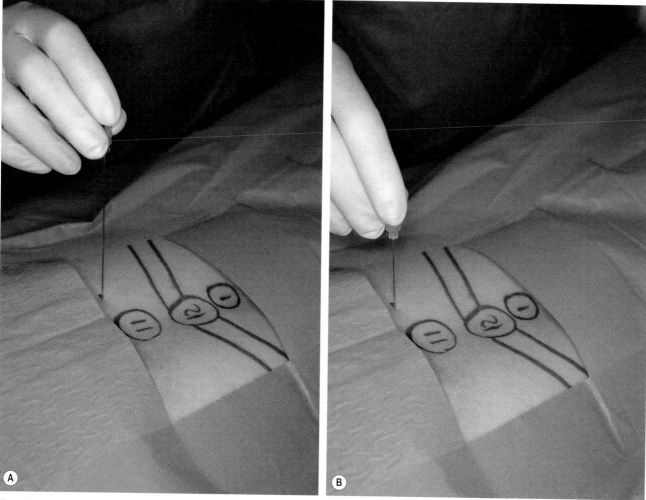

Fig. 4.4.4

- After further aspiration, lidocaine (lignocaine) 1% 0.1–1 ml is injected.
- After 5 minutes the patient is questioned about changes in pain and sensation in the distribution of the nerve root.
- For diagnostic nerve root blockade the needle may be removed when the level causing pain is identified.

Confirmation of a successful block

- Relief of pain and anesthesia in distribution of the blocked nerve.

Tips

- An alternative approach is to advance the needle in a mesiad direction until the lamina is contacted. The needle is inserted more medially, 1.5 cm lateral to the cephalad edge of the spinous process and then walked laterally off the edge of the lamina until it slips into the costovertebral ligament and is advanced 1 cm.

- Some workers advocate applying an air-filled loss-of-resistance syringe to the needle after it has been walked off the transverse process or lamina, and advancing the needle while applying pressure to the plunger. Loss of resistance has been described as the needle pops through the costotransverse ligament to enter the thoracic paravertebral space.
- A catheter may be passed into the paravertebral space via an epidural needle, with the bevel medial, by using this technique.

Potential problems

- Pneumothorax.
- While it has been recommended that the needle be angled 20° medially after entering the paravertebral space, care must be taken with the aid of fluoroscopy that the local anesthetic solution is not injected into the nerve sheath causing the solution to track centrally to produce intrathecal blockade.

- Epidural blockade usually occurs with this block, but this is not a problem once low volumes are used. However, even small volumes of epidural spread may confound the diagnostic value of the block.
- Sympathetic blockade may cause hemodynamic changes.
- Neuritis may occur with catheter placement.

- Intravascular injection. Injection of particulate steroids into a radicular artery can cause spinal cord infarction. Particulate steroids should never be injected near the foramen unless intravascular placement has been ruled out using live fluoroscopy contrast dye injection, preferably with digital subtraction technique.

4.5 SACRAL NERVE ROOT BLOCK

Anatomy

Each of the five sacral nerves is accessible by passing a needle into the sacral foramen via the posterior opening at the level of the nerve. The sacral canal is the caudal extension of the epidural space and nerves of the cauda equina leave via the sacral foramina (**Fig. 4.5.1**). The distal dural sac ends at S2, the level of the posterior superior iliac spines. The epidural space ends at the sacral hiatus (**Fig. 4.5.2**). While variability in the bony anatomy of the sacrum is common, this occurs usually in the midline.

Equipment

- 2 ml and 10 ml syringes
- 25 G needle
- 22 G spinal needle, end-opening
- ECG, BP, and SpO$_2$ monitors
- Resuscitation equipment (*see Appendix 3*) and drugs
- Fluoroscopy or ultrasound

Drugs

- Lidocaine (lignocaine) 1% 10 ml (or its equivalent)
- Corticosteroid if indicated, e.g. triamcinolone diacetate 50 mg (or its equivalent)
- Resuscitation drugs (*see Appendix 3*)

Position of patient

- Prone.
- Pillow under anterior superior iliac spine to flatten the normal lumbar lordosis (*Fig. 4.5.3*).

Needle puncture and technique

- Intravenous access is inserted.
- Monitors are attached.
- Resuscitation equipment and drugs are checked and made ready for use.
- The sacral midline and an area 10 cm × 5 cm laterally is cleaned with antiseptic solution and a fenestrated drape is placed over the sterile area.

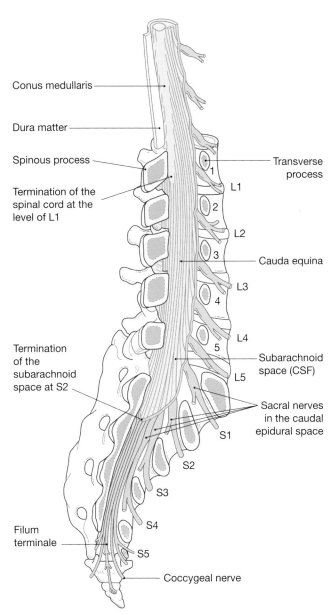

Fig. 4.5.1

Conus medullaris

Dura matter

Spinous process

Termination of the spinal cord at the level of L1

Transverse process

Cauda equina

Subarachnoid space (CSF)

Termination of the subarachnoid space at S2

Sacral nerves in the caudal epidural space

Filum terminale

Coccygeal nerve

L1
L2
L3
L4
L5
S1
S2
S3
S4
S5

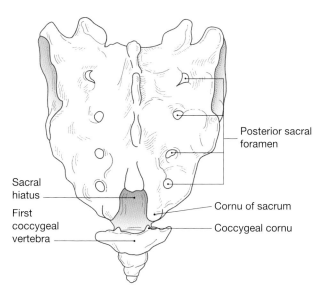

Fig. 4.5.2

Posterior sacral foramen

Sacral hiatus

First coccygeal vertebra

Cornu of sacrum

Coccygeal cornu

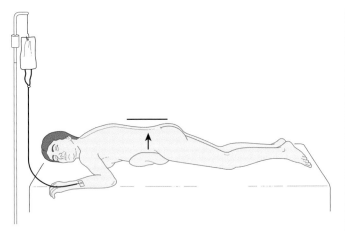

Fig. 4.5.3

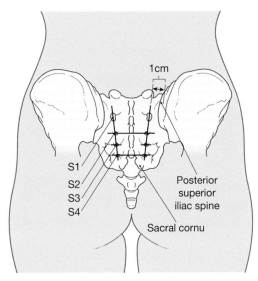

Fig. 4.5.4

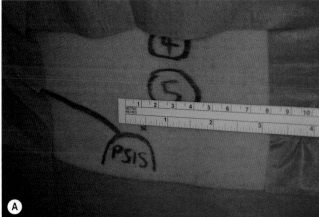

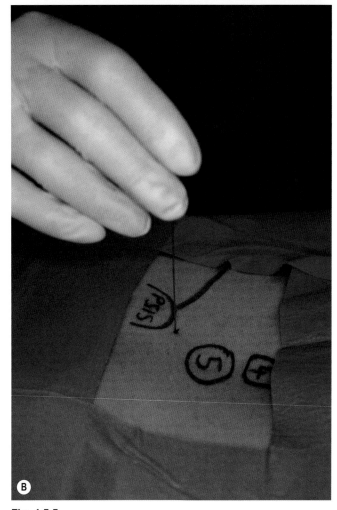

Fig. 4.5.5

- Iliac crests are palpated and an intercrestal line is identified.
- This corresponds with the inferior aspect of the spinous process of L4 or may lie in the L4–5 interspace.
- For this block, it is almost essential that the posterior opening of the sacral foramina is identified with fluoroscopy. The X-ray beam is used to guide the needle tip into the foramen. It is important to note that when the anteroposterior X-ray view is used, it is usually the anterior opening of the foramen that is the most prominent.
- **The insertion point of the needle lies 2–3 cm lateral to the midline (variable) and approximately 1 cm medial to the posterior iliac spine** (*Figs 4.5.4, 4.5.5 a,b*).
- Therefore, with the aid of fluoroscopy, the insertion point is identified.
- A skin wheal is raised and the area is infiltrated with lidocaine (lignocaine) 1%.

- A spinal needle is introduced in a vertical direction to the skin, and aimed slightly cephalad until bone is contacted (*Fig. 4.5.6*).
- The needle is then walked off the sacrum in a caudad direction until it slips into the foramen. After confirmation with the aid of fluoroscopy it is then advanced 1 cm.

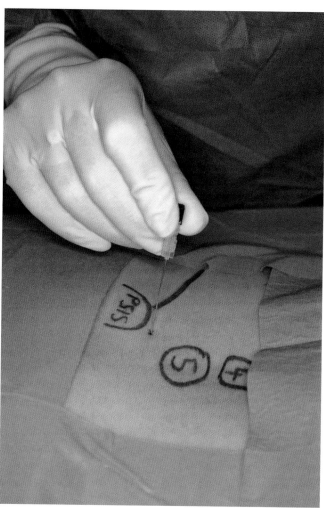

Fig. 4.5.6

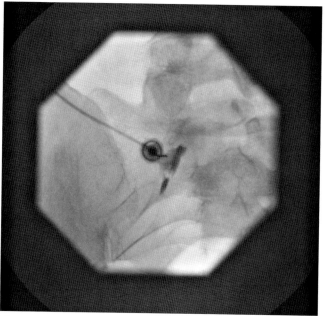

Fig. 4.5.7

- Paresthesia may be produced.
- After aspiration, non-ionic radio-opaque contrast medium 0.5 ml is injected.
- The correct placement is indicated by a needle tip flush with the anterior surface of the spinal canal in the lateral fluoroscopic view.
- Injection of 0.5 ml non-ionic contrast should spread diagonally along the S1 spinal nerve (*Fig. 4.5.7*).
- After further aspiration, lidocaine (lignocaine) 1% 0.5 ml is injected.
- After 5 minutes, the patient is questioned about changes in pain, sensation and power of the lower limb.
- For diagnostic nerve root blockade the needle may be removed when the level causing pain is identified.
- Ultrasound may also aid placement.

Confirmation of a successful block

- Relief of pain.
- Anesthesia in the distribution of the blocked nerve.

Tips

- Some workers advocate drawing a line from a point 2–3 cm medial to the posterior superior iliac spine to a point 1–2 cm lateral to the sacral cornua. The sacral foramina usually lie along this line.
- It is best to angle the X-ray beam caudally, thereby perpendicular to the sacrum, superimposing the anterior and posterior sacral foramina. Consequently, when the needle is introduced in a direction perpendicular (*Fig. 4.5.8*) to the skin, fluoroscopic guidance is easier. Optimally, the needle makes gentle contact with the spinal nerve in the middle of the canal (*Figs 4.5.9, 4.5.10*) and produces paresthesia in the distribution of the nerve.
- While all sacral nerve roots are accessible, using this technique for blockade of S5 is achieved by walking the needle caudally off the inferior edge of the bony plate of the sacrum and advancing the needle 1 cm.

Potential problems

- Caudal epidural blockade may occur with this block, but this is not a problem once low volumes are used. However, even small volumes of epidural spread may confound the diagnostic value of the block.
- Intravascular injection. Injection of particulate steroids into a radicular artery can cause spinal cord infarction. Particulate steroids should never be injected near the foramen unless intravascular placement has been ruled out using live fluoroscopy contrast dye injection, preferably with digital subtraction technique.

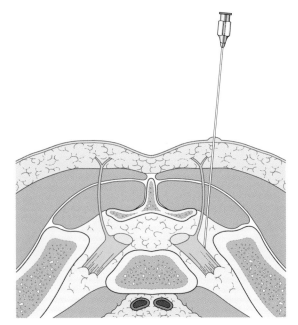

Fig. 4.5.8

Fig. 4.5.9

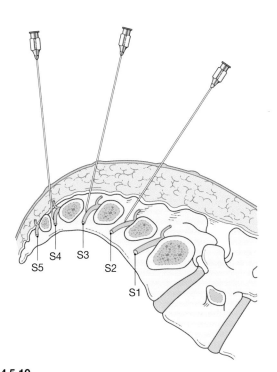

Fig. 4.5.10

4.6 OCCIPITAL NERVE BLOCK

Anatomy

The greater occipital nerve arises from the dorsal rami of the second cervical nerve. From here it passes through the muscles of the neck and becomes subcutaneous at the superior nuchal line, where it emerges with the occipital artery (Fig. 4.6.1). The superior nuchal line extends from the mastoid process to the greater occipital protuberance bilaterally (Fig. 4.6.2).

Equipment

- 10 ml syringe
- 25 G needle

- ECG, BP, and SpO$_2$ monitors
- Resuscitation equipment (*see Appendix 3*)

Drugs

- Lidocaine (lignocaine) 1% 10 ml (or its equivalent)
- Corticosteroid if indicated, e.g. triamcinolone diacetate 50 mg (or its equivalent)
- Resuscitation drugs (*see Appendix 3*)

Position of patient

- Sitting.
- Neck flexed.

Needle puncture and technique

- The superior nuchal line is cleaned with antiseptic solution (no drape is required) (*Fig. 4.6.3*).

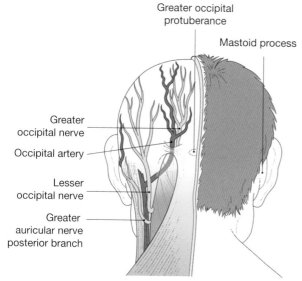

Greater occipital protuberance

Mastoid process

Greater occipital nerve

Occipital artery

Lesser occipital nerve

Greater auricular nerve posterior branch

Fig. 4.6.1

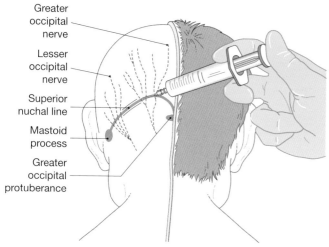

Greater occipital nerve

Lesser occipital nerve

Superior nuchal line

Mastoid process

Greater occipital protuberance

Fig. 4.6.2

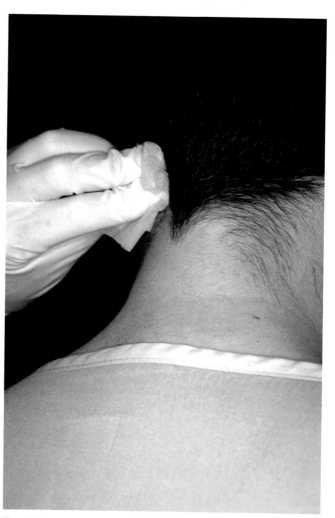

Fig. 4.6.3

- The occipital artery is palpated 2 cm lateral to the greater occipital protuberance on the superior nuchal line (*Fig. 4.6.4*).
- A 25 G needle is inserted subcutaneously at this point.
- After negative aspiration, 3–5 ml of lidocaine (lignocaine) 1% or its equivalent, plus corticosteroid if indicated, is injected to surround the occipital artery.
- It is often difficult to feel an occipital artery pulse. If this is the case, it is best to pick a point midway between the occipital protuberance and the mastoid bone and fan out the injection in both directions, medially and laterally from that site (*Fig. 4.6.5*).

Confirmation of a successful block

- Relief of pain and anesthesia in distribution of nerve.

Tips

- Bone should be contacted at a depth no greater than 1–2 cm.
- The lesser occipital nerve is blocked by redirecting the needle towards the mastoid process along the greater nuchal line and injecting a further 3 ml of solution.

Potential problems

- Injection into the cerebrospinal fluid (CSF) of the cisterna magna is possible and will produce a total spinal block.

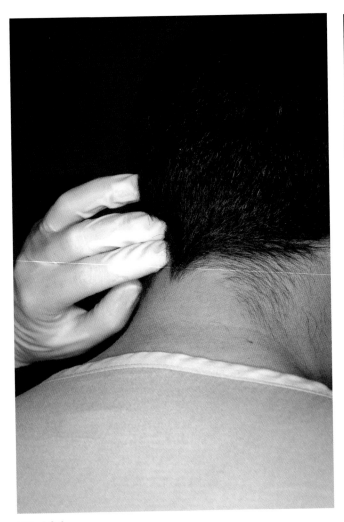

Fig. 4.6.4

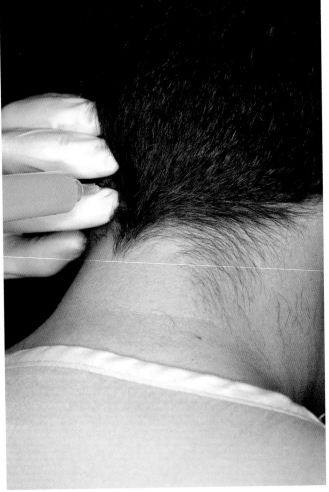

Fig. 4.6.5

4.7 TRIGEMINAL GANGLION (GASSERIAN) BLOCK

Anatomy

The trigeminal ganglion gives rise to the fifth cranial nerve and divides into three branches, the ophthalmic, maxillary, and mandibular nerves (Fig. 4.7.1). These provide the sensory nerve supply to the ipsilateral face and the anterior two-thirds of the head (Fig. 4.7.2). The mandibular nerve also provides motor supply to the muscles of mastication.

The trigeminal ganglion is located at the apex of the petrous temporal bone in a fold of dura mater, "Meckel's cave". This dural invagination covers the posterior two-thirds of the ganglion and contains cerebrospinal fluid (CSF). Posterior to Meckel's cave lies the brainstem, superior to it lies the temporal lobe, and medially lies the cavernous sinus which contains the internal carotid artery and cranial nerves III, IV, and VI. Accordingly, extreme care must be taken when carrying out this block, especially if neurolytic agents are used. Blockade of the ganglion is carried out by passage of a needle through the foramen ovale, which lies immediately below it (Fig. 4.7.3).

Equipment

- 2 ml and 10 ml syringes
- 25 G needle
- 22 G 8–10 cm needle
- Non-ionic radio-opaque contrast medium
- ECG, BP, and SpO_2 monitors
- Resuscitation equipment (*see Appendix 3*)
- Fluoroscopy

Drugs

- Lidocaine (lignocaine) 2% 10 ml
- Lidocaine (lignocaine) 1% 10 ml (or its equivalent)
- Neurolytic agent, e.g. phenol 6% plus glycerol (or its equivalent)
- Sedative, e.g. midazolam, propofol
- Resuscitation drugs (*see Appendix 3*)

Position of patient

- Supine.
- Eyes directed straight ahead.

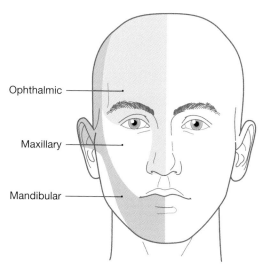

Ophthalmic

Maxillary

Mandibular

Fig. 4.7.1

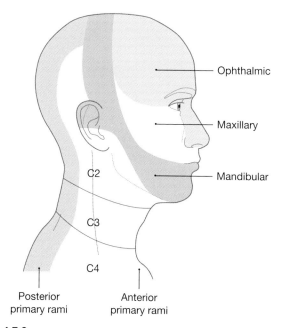

Ophthalmic

Maxillary

Mandibular

C2

C3

C4

Posterior primary rami

Anterior primary rami

Fig. 4.7.2

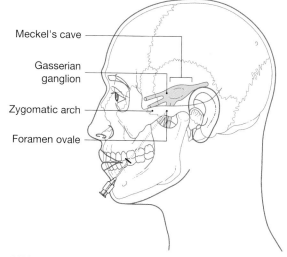

Meckel's cave

Gasserian ganglion

Zygomatic arch

Foramen ovale

Fig. 4.7.3

Needle puncture and technique

Caution: Injection of 0.25 ml of lidocaine (lignocaine) 1% into the CSF may result in immediate convulsion and/or loss of consciousness with possible cardiovascular system (CVS) collapse.

- The cheek on the side of the block is cleaned with antiseptic solution or saline.
- Mild sedation is induced.
- It is best to stand on the side of the block, just below the shoulder.
- **The insertion point lies 1–3 cm posterior to the lateral margin of the mouth, at the medial edge of the masseter muscle (located by asking the patient to clench the jaw) and is marked.**
- **In edentulous patients the insertion point should be more caudad** as sufficient angle towards the infratemporal surface of the sphenoid bone may not be achieved.
- One finger is placed inside the upper lip to avoid injection into the buccal cavity and possible bacterial contamination, and a skin wheal is raised at this site.
- Viewed from above, a 22 G 8–10 cm needle is advanced towards the ipsilateral pupil (*Figs 4.7.4–4.7.6*), or viewed from the side the needle advances towards the mid-point of the zygomatic arch (see Anatomy above) until bone is contacted; the roof of the infratemporal fossa. This lies just anterior to the foramen ovale and lateral to the base of the pterygoid process. The location of the needle tip is confirmed with fluoroscopy.
- A depth mark is set and the needle is withdrawn to the subcutaneous tissue. With the aid of fluoroscopy

the needle is reinserted to walk off the bone and enter the foramen ovale (*Fig. 4.7.7*).

- Paresthesia in the distribution of the mandibular nerve (sometimes the other branches of the trigeminal nerve) or contraction of the muscles of mastication may be experienced at this point.
- The needle is advanced a further 1 cm to bring the tip to lie in the trigeminal ganglion. The correct placement is indicated by a visible outline of Meckel's cave on injection of 0.25 ml non-ionic radio-opaque contrast medium under fluoroscopy (*Figs 4.7.8, 4.7.9*).
- The patient is allowed to awaken from sedation and is questioned about the presence and distribution of paresthesia and pain.
- A stimulating device may aid placement in patients who are not able to locate the paresthesia with accuracy.
- If necessary, analgesia may be administered, although this may affect accurate assessment of the blockade.
- Adjustment of the needle may be required to place the needle near the appropriate nerve division.

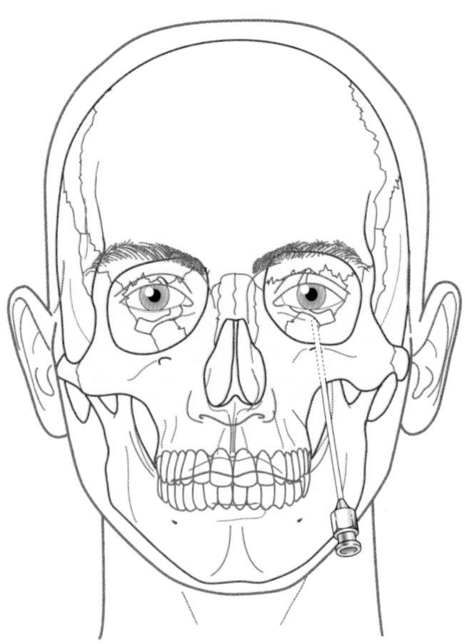

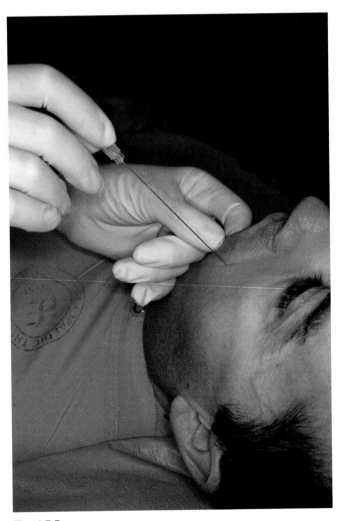

Fig. 4.7.4

Fig. 4.7.5

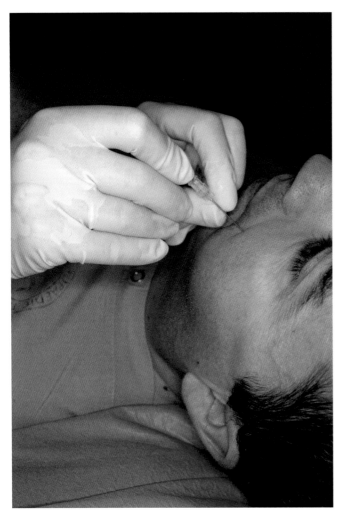

Fig. 4.7.6

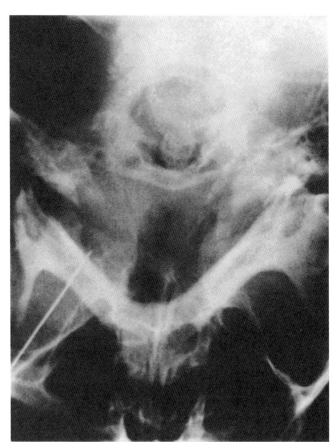

Fig. 4.7.8

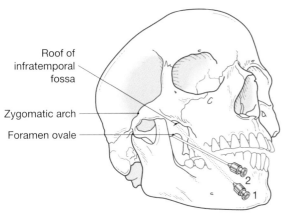

Roof of
infratemporal
fossa

Zygomatic arch

Foramen ovale

Fig. 4.7.7

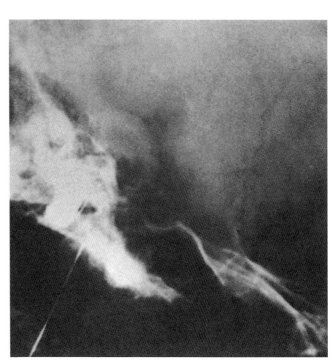

Fig. 4.7.9

- After careful negative aspiration for CSF or blood, lidocaine (lignocaine) 1% 0.25 ml is injected (*Caution: injection into CSF may cause loss of consciousness.*) This is followed by further boluses of lidocaine (lignocaine) 1% 0.25 ml until a total of 1 ml is given.
- After 5 minutes the patient is questioned about pain relief and changes in sensation.
- When the desired analgesia has been achieved for diagnostic blockade the needle may be removed.

Confirmation of a successful block

- Relief of pain and anesthesia in the distribution of the trigeminal nerve or its desired branches.

Tips

- Intravenous anesthesia using a short-acting agent, e.g. propofol, may be induced to allow placement of the needle. The patient is then allowed to awaken and a stimulating device may aid accurate placement of the needle.
- The needle is advanced beyond the infratemporal bone by 0.5 cm for location of the mandibular division, 1.0 cm for the maxillary division, and 1.5 cm for the ophthalmic division.

- Gangliolysis using thermocoagulation may be employed for trigeminal-nerve division destruction after location of the ganglion using this technique. Further intravenous anesthesia using a short-acting agent, e.g. propofol, may be induced after placement of the insulated needle to facilitate this painful procedure.
- Injection of glycerol alone may produce pain relief with this injection technique. This involves placement of the needle in the cul-de-sac of CSF, positioning the patient face-down or supine, with the head extended to prevent spill-over into the posterior cranial fossa. After entry into the CSF, and positive aspiration of CSF, 0.1–0.3 ml of glycerol may be injected.

Potential problems

- Injection of 0.25 ml of lidocaine (lignocaine) 1% into the CSF may result in immediate convulsion and/or loss of consciousness with possible CVS collapse.
- Spread of hyperbaric neurolytic solution may immediately affect cranial nerves VI, VIII, IX, X, XI, and XII.
- Spread of hypobaric neurolytic solution may immediately affect the oculomotor and trochlear nerves.
- Neurolytic blocks of the trigeminal ganglion commonly produce corneal and hemifacial anesthesia.

AUTONOMIC BLOCKADE 5

Autonomic blockade is useful in the diagnosis and treatment of pain of autonomic origin. In cases of thoracic, abdominal or pelvic pain, it is often difficult to distinguish between that of visceral origin and that of somatic. Pain of visceral origin, e.g. pancreatic cancer or pelvic cancer, may cause pain that responds to celiac or hypogastric plexus blockade, respectively. A prognostic block may be carried out prior to neurolytic blockade for relief of cancer pain. Pain of the upper abdominal viscera may also be relieved by celiac plexus block, proceeding to neurolytic blockade as appropriate for cancer-related pain. The retrocrural approach to the celiac plexus also targets the splanchnic nerves to produce a splanchnic nerve block if required. Chest pain may be of somatic origin, e.g. intercostal neuralgia and costochondritis, or visceral origin, e.g. pulmonary or cardiac-related pain. Stellate ganglion blockade may be helpful in the diagnosis and management of the latter.

In addition, increased sympathetic activity is thought to contribute to a large number of pain states. These are generally grouped under the term Complex Regional Pain Syndrome Type I and II. In these cases, trophic changes and alterations in blood flow are often obvious but the pathophysiologic origin is not. Blockade of sympathetic innervation may therefore help in diagnosis and management of such pain. This may also indicate other therapies that could be beneficial, e.g. sympathetically active drugs or destructive therapies. Similarly, these therapies would not be indicated if sympathetic blockade failed to relieve the pain. If blockade did succeed in relieving this type of pain, further blocks may effect lasting relief.

There are a number of other conditions in which the diagnosis is clear but there is a possible contribution of sympathetic activity in the pathogenesis of the pain. These conditions include central pain, post-herpetic neuralgia, trigeminal neuralgia, peripheral vascular disease and others. Blockade of sympathetic activity may help to clarify the sympathetic contribution to the pain and therefore help to indicate management options.

5.1 STELLATE GANGLION BLOCK—C6 (CLASSIC) APPROACH

Anatomy

The cervical sympathetic trunk—the superior, middle, and stellate ganglia—supplies the sympathetic innervation of the head, neck, and upper limbs. The stellate ganglion is made up of a combination of the lower cervical and first thoracic ganglia. It lies on the prevertebral fascia of the seventh cervical and first thoracic vertebrae (Fig. 5.1.1). However, as the sixth cervical anterior tubercle (Chassaignac's tubercle) is easy to palpate, injection of a large volume of local anesthetic is made at this level and allowed to track caudally along the prevertebral fascia to block the stellate ganglion. The vertebral and carotid arteries, the pleura, and the brachial plexus are in close proximity to the stellate ganglion.

Equipment

- 10 ml syringe
- 22 G short-bevel needle
- Extension set (optional)
- ECG, BP, SpO$_2$ monitors
- Skin temperature monitor
- Resuscitation equipment (see Appendix 3)
- Ultrasound (optional)

Drugs

- Lidocaine (lignocaine) 1%, 10 ml
- Resuscitation drugs (see Appendix 3)

Position of patient

- Supine.
- Thin pillow under head.
- Roll under neck.
- Eyes directed at ceiling.
- Mouth slightly open.

Needle puncture and technique

Caution: Injection of 0.5–1 ml of lidocaine (lignocaine) 1% into the vertebral artery may result in immediate convulsion and/or loss of consciousness with possible cardiovascular system (CVS) collapse.

- Intravenous access is inserted.
- Monitors are attached, each temperature probe is attached to the palmar aspect of the middle finger of each hand (*Fig. 5.1.2*).
- Resuscitation equipment and drugs are checked and made ready for use.
- The side of the neck is cleaned with antiseptic solution.
- It is best to stand at the same side of the neck as the ganglion to be blocked.

FOR THE RIGHT-HANDED OPERATOR

With the left hand
- The thyroid cartilage is located and marked.
- The cricoid cartilage is identified and marked (*Figs 5.1.3, 5.1.4*).

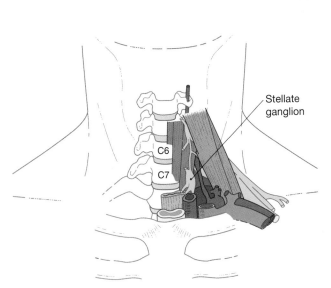

Stellate ganglion

C6

C7

Fig. 5.1.1

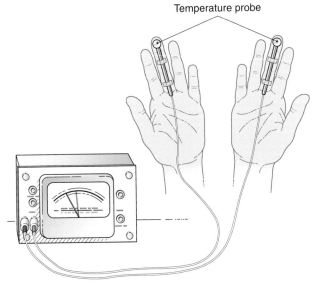

Temperature probe

Fig. 5.1.2

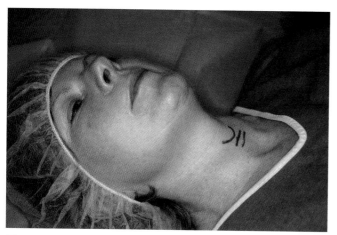

Fig. 5.1.3

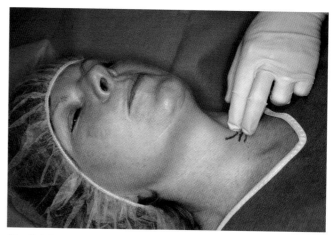

Fig. 5.1.6

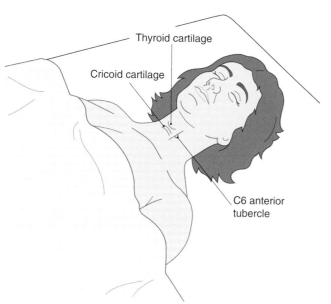

Thyroid cartilage

Cricoid cartilage

C6 anterior
tubercle

Fig. 5.1.4

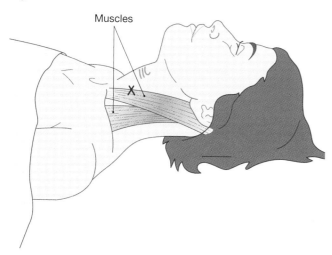

Muscles

Fig. 5.1.5

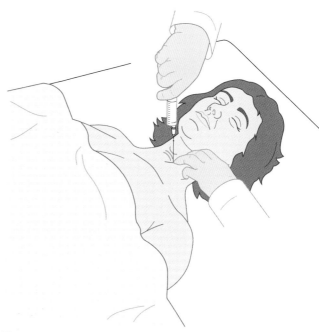

Fig. 5.1.7

- Chassaignac's tubercle is palpated with the middle finger, just lateral to the cricoid cartilage (*Fig. 5.1.5*).
- The sternocleidomastoid (SCM) muscle is gently pulled laterally and the carotid pulse is palpated (*Fig. 5.1.6*).
- Chassaignac's tubercle is palpated again and positioned between the fore- and middle fingers.

With the right hand
- The needle is inserted between the fore- and middle fingers of the other hand, directly perpendicular to the floor, aiming for Chassaignac's tubercle (*Figs 5.1.7, 5.1.8*).
- When contact with the tubercle is reached, the injecting hand is steadied and the needle is withdrawn 2 mm.
- The hub of the needle is held in place with the other hand.

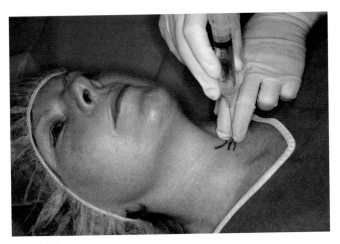

Fig. 5.1.8

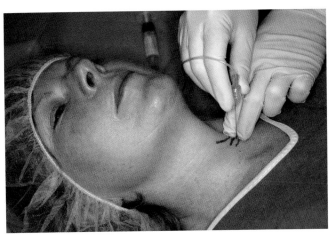

Fig. 5.1.9

- After negative aspiration, lidocaine (lignocaine) 1%, 0.5 ml, is injected.
- The patient is questioned about sensation and any change in level of consciousness is noted.
- If negative, the same procedure is repeated as 0.5 ml boluses are given until 10 ml is injected.
- The needle is withdrawn and the patient is immediately put in the sitting position.
- Monitors should be left attached and i.v. access left in situ for at least 30 minutes. The patient is requested not to eat or drink for 2 hours, as the recurrent laryngeal nerve may be blocked.
- Note: if aspiration of blood occurs during the block the needle is removed and cleared, keeping left fore- and middle fingers in place. It is then reinserted and the block is continued as above.
- If hematoma occurs before the solution is injected it may be worth performing the block at the C7 level.
- If there is pain on injection and/or paresthesia, it is likely that the brachial plexus may have been contacted, the needle is withdrawn and the landmarks are rechecked.

Confirmation of a successful block

- Skin temperature, measured over the palmar aspect of the hand or fingers on the blocked side, should begin to rise within 2–3 minutes. Extensive sympathetic blockade is confirmed by a rise in skin temperature to >33 °C.
- Ptosis of eyelid.
- Miosis of pupil.
- Unilateral blockage of nose on side of block.
- Unilateral flushing of conjunctiva of eye on side of block.

- Blockade of the upper sympathetic chain can occur in the absence of sympathetic denervation of the upper extremity, resulting in Horner's syndrome without a rise in skin temperature in the hand.

Tips

- The external jugular vein usually crosses the SCM muscle at the level of C6.
- Skin infiltration prior to block should be avoided if possible, as this will make landmarks more difficult to locate.
- If palpation is painful or difficult it may be helpful to try to bounce the middle finger off the tubercle during identification.
- An extension set may be inserted between the needle and syringe for better stability of needle (*Fig. 5.1.9*), but an assistant is then required to continue the procedure as described above.
- Consideration should be given to performance of the block under fluoroscopy or CT control if the landmarks are difficult to locate.
- Lidocaine (lignocaine) 1% 15 ml may be given if a previous block failed to relieve sympathetically maintained pain in the presence of correctly placed solution. This may improve tracking of the solution caudally to produce more effective blockade of the stellate ganglion.
- Ultrasound may aid placement of needle (*Fig. 5.1.10 a,b*).

Potential problems

- Intra-arterial injection or intrathecal injection may result in immediate convulsion and/or loss of consciousness with possible CVS collapse.

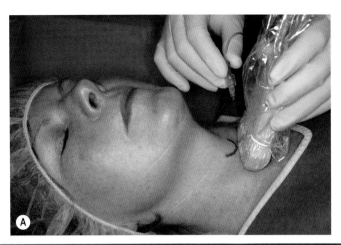

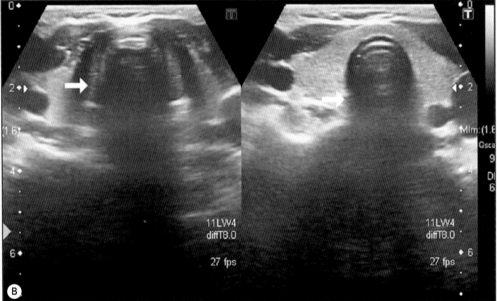

Fig. 5.1.10 From Gupta Prashant K, Gupta Kumkum, Dwivedi Amit Nandan D, Jain Manish. Potential role of ultrasound in anesthesia and intensive care, Anesthesia Essays and Research, 2011 Volume 5, Issue Number 1, Page: 11-19.

- Hematoma may occur (avoid performing block on patients who have coagulopathy).
- Pneumothorax may occur.
- Recurrent laryngeal nerve block may occur and it is prudent to advise the patient about possible hoarseness post-blockade. Bilateral stellate ganglion blockade should be avoided for the same reason.
- Phrenic nerve block may occur and it is prudent to caution the patient about possible shortness of breath post blockade of the stellate ganglion.

5.2 STELLATE GANGLION BLOCK—C7 APPROACH

Anatomy

As for stellate ganglion block (C6 approach) in Section 5.1 (Figs 5.2.1 a,b).

Equipment

- 10 ml syringe
- 22 G short-bevel needle
- Extension set (optional)
- ECG, BP, SpO$_2$ monitors
- Skin temperature monitor
- Fluoroscopy or CT (optional)
- Resuscitation equipment (*see Appendix 3*)
- Ultrasound (optional)

Drugs

- Lidocaine (lignocaine) 1%, 10 ml
- Resuscitation drugs (*see Appendix 3*)

Position of patient

- Supine.
- Thin pillow under head.
- Roll under neck.
- Eyes directed at ceiling.
- Mouth slightly open.

Needle puncture and technique

Caution: injection of 0.5–1 ml of lidocaine (lignocaine) 1% into the vertebral artery may result in immediate convulsion and/or loss of consciousness with possible cardiovascular (CVS) collapse. The risk of pneumothorax is greater with this approach.

- Intravenous access is inserted.
- Monitors are attached.
- Each temperature probe is attached to the palmar aspect of the middle finger of each hand. (*Fig. 5.2.2*).
- Resuscitation equipment and drugs are checked and made ready for use.
- The side of the neck is cleaned with antiseptic solution.

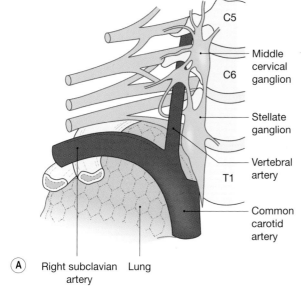

(A) Right subclavian artery   Lung

Labels: C5, Middle cervical ganglion, C6, Stellate ganglion, Vertebral artery, T1, Common carotid artery

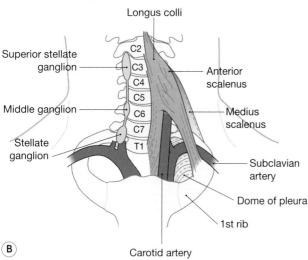

(B)

Labels: Longus colli, Superior stellate ganglion, C2, C3, Anterior scalenus, C4, C5, Middle ganglion, C6, Medius scalenus, C7, Stellate ganglion, T1, Subclavian artery, Dome of pleura, 1st rib, Carotid artery

Fig. 5.2.1

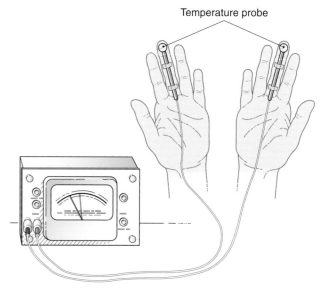

Temperature probe

Fig. 5.2.2

- It is best to stand at the same side of the neck as the ganglion to be blocked.

FOR THE RIGHT-HANDED OPERATOR

With the left hand

- The thyroid cartilage is located and marked.
- The cricoid cartilage is identified and marked (*Figs 5.2.3, 5.2.4*).
- The sternoclavicular junction is palpated and marked (*Fig. 5.2.5*).
- The SCM muscle is gently pulled laterally and the carotid pulse is palpated (*Fig. 5.2.6*).
- **The site of insertion of the needle lies 3 cm above the sternoclavicular junction or one to two finger-breadths below the level of the cricoid cartilage.**

With the right hand

- The patient is requested to exhale deeply before needle insertion to minimize the risk of pneumothorax.
- The needle is inserted between the fore- and middle fingers of the other hand, directly perpendicular to the floor.
- When contact with the transverse process of C7 is reached, the injecting hand is steadied and the needle is withdrawn 2 mm.
- The hub of the needle is held in place with the other hand.
- After negative aspiration, lidocaine (lignocaine) 1%, 0.5 ml, is injected.
- The patient is questioned about sensation, and any change in level of consciousness is noted.
- If negative, the same procedure is repeated and 0.5 ml boluses are given until 5–8 ml is injected.
- The needle is withdrawn and the patient is immediately put in the sitting position.

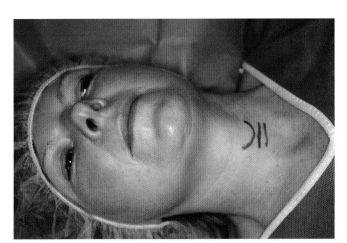

Fig. 5.2.3

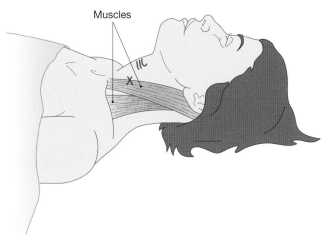

Fig. 5.2.5

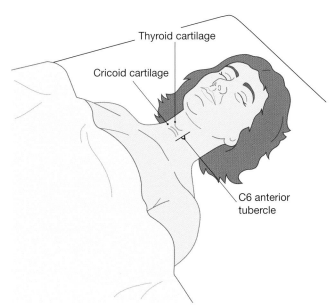

Fig. 5.2.4

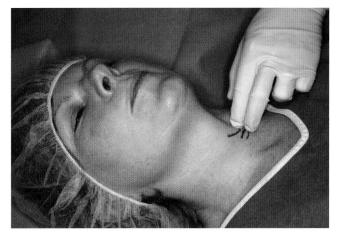

Fig. 5.2.6

- Monitors should be left attached and i.v. access left in situ for at least 30 minutes. Blockade of the recurrent laryngeal nerve is less likely with the C7 approach but it is wise to advise the patient not to eat or drink for 2 hours.
- Note: if aspiration of blood occurs during the block, the needle is removed and cleared, keeping the left fore- and middle fingers in place. It is then reinserted and the block is continued as above.
- If there is pain on injection and/or paresthesia, it is likely that the brachial plexus may have been contacted, the needle is withdrawn and the landmarks are rechecked.
- Ultrasound may aid placement of the needle.

Confirmation of a successful block

- Temperature increase >1° on the side of block. The temperature should begin to rise in the finger of the blocked side within 3 minutes of injection.
- Ptosis of eyelid.
- Miosis of pupil.
- Unilateral blockage of nose on side of block.
- Unilateral flushing of conjunctiva of eye on side of block.
- Relief of sympathetically maintained pain.

Tips

- Some workers advocate targeting the **ventrolateral aspect of the C7 vertebral body instead of its transverse process**. The needle is directed 15–20° medially. With the aid of fluoroscopy, ultrasound or CT, the vertebral body is contacted just medial to the insertion of the longus colli muscle. The needle is then withdrawn

2 mm, stabilized, and 1 ml of non-ionic contrast medium is injected.
- The external jugular vein usually crosses the SCM muscle at the level of C6.
- Skin infiltration prior to block should be avoided if possible, as this will make landmarks more difficult to locate.
- An extension set may be inserted between the needle and syringe for better stability of needle, but an assistant is then required to continue the procedure as described above.
- Lidocaine (lignocaine) 1% 10 ml may be given if a previous block failed to relieve sympathetically maintained pain in the presence of correctly placed solution. This may improve tracking of the solution caudally to produce more effective blockade of the stellate ganglion.

Potential problems

- Intra-arterial injection or intrathecal injection may result in immediate convulsion and/or loss of consciousness with possible CVS collapse.
- Hematoma may occur (avoid performing block on patients who have coagulopathy).
- Pneumothorax may occur (more likely with C7 approach).
- Recurrent laryngeal nerve block may occur and it is prudent to advise the patient about possible hoarseness post blockade. Bilateral stellate ganglion blockade should be avoided for the same reason.
- Phrenic nerve block may occur and it is prudent to caution the patient about possible shortness of breath following blockade of the stellate ganglion.

5.3 LUMBAR SYMPATHETIC BLOCK

Anatomy

The lumbar sympathetic chain is located in the prevertebral fascia, which lies on the anterolateral aspects of the vertebral bodies. The psoas muscle separates the lumbar sympathetic chain from the lumbar somatic nerves. A single injection of local anesthetic at the level of L2 will usually provide a complete block of postganglionic sympathetic efferents to the lower extremity because the lowest preganglionic sympathetic outflow to the chain is at the level of L2.

Equipment

- 2 ml, 5 ml, and 10 ml syringes
- 30 G needle
- Two 15 cm 22 G needles
- Extension set (optional)
- ECG, BP, SpO₂ monitors
- Skin temperature monitor (two probes)
- Resuscitation equipment (see Appendix 3)
- Fluoroscopy

Drugs

- Lidocaine (lignocaine) 1%, 5 ml for skin infiltration
- Lidocaine (lignocaine) 1%, 15–20 ml (or its equivalent) for block
- Phenol 6%
- Radio-opaque contrast medium
- Resuscitation drugs (see Appendix 3)

Position of patient

- Prone.
- Pillow under anterior superior iliac spine to flatten the normal lumbar lordosis (Fig. 5.3.1).

Needle puncture and technique

- Intravenous access is inserted.
- Monitors are attached.
- Each temperature probe is attached to the plantar aspect of the big toe (Fig. 5.3.2).
- Resuscitation equipment and drugs are checked and made ready for use.
- The thoracolumbar midline and an area 10 cm × 5 cm laterally is cleaned with antiseptic solution and a fenestrated drape is placed over the sterile area.
- The twelfth rib is identified and a line is drawn along its inferior border (Fig. 5.3.3 a,b).
- The iliac crests are palpated and the intercrestal line is identified (this corresponds with the inferior aspect of the spinous process of L4 or may lie in the L4–5 interspace).
- The spinous processes are counted until L2 is identified and confirmed with fluoroscopy.
- **The insertion point lies 8 cm lateral to the L2 spinous process and is also marked** (Fig. 5.3.4).
- A skin wheal is raised at one of the marked sites and the area is infiltrated with lidocaine (lignocaine) 1%.
- At a 30° angle to the frontal plane, a 22 G 15 cm needle is advanced slightly cephalad towards the lower

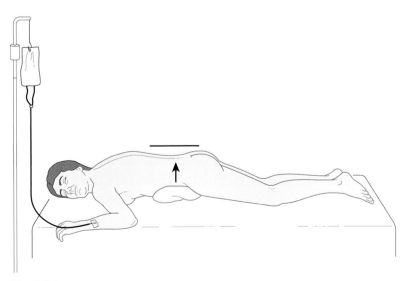

Fig. 5.3.1

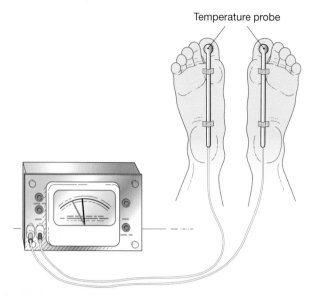

Temperature probe

Fig. 5.3.2

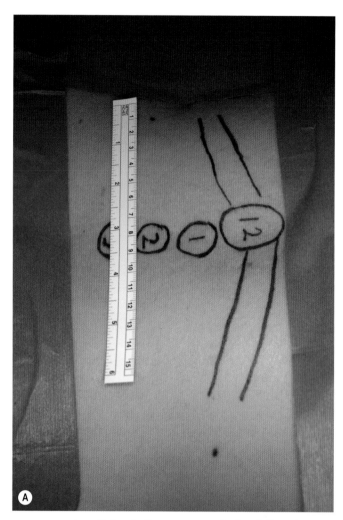

portion of the L2 vertebral body (*Fig. 5.3.5*), until its vertebral body is contacted at a depth of about 7–9 cm and confirmed with fluoroscopy. If the needle contacts bone at a more superficial level, it is probable that it has come into contact with the transverse process and it will need to be repositioned.

- The needle depth is noted.
- The needle is then withdrawn to the subcutaneous tissue and, with the aid of fluoroscopy, it is re-advanced, this time at an angle 45° to the frontal plane, until the previous depth (as noted) is reached. It should slip past the vertebral body at a depth about 1–2 cm deeper than the first depth mark (*Fig. 5.3.6*).
- After negative aspiration, the fluoroscopic image is observed as a small amount of non-ionic radio-contrast medium is injected. The correct placement of the needle is indicated by the presence of a layer of contrast medium in a thin line along the anterior border of the vertebral column (*Figs 5.3.7–5.3.9*).
- After further negative aspirations, 5 ml of lidocaine (lignocaine) 1% is injected. The patient is questioned about pain relief and observations of skin temperature are made. There should be little resistance to injection, similar to resistance felt when injecting through an epidural needle. If resistance is encountered, or if the injection is painful, the needle should be repositioned. A unilateral rise in skin temperature indicates a successful block.
- After 10 minutes the patient is questioned about pain relief and any symptoms of somatic nerve blockade. Sensory and motor functioning of the lower extremities is checked. The procedure should be abandoned if there is evidence of somatic blockade.

Ⓐ

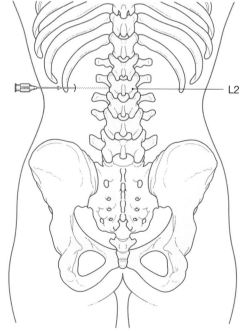

L2

Ⓑ

Fig. 5.3.3

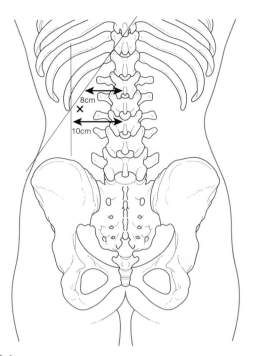

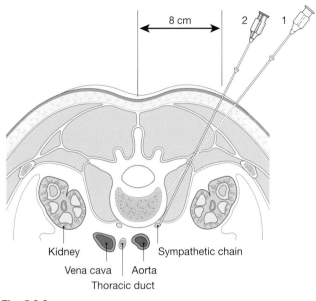

Fig. 5.3.6

Fig. 5.3.4

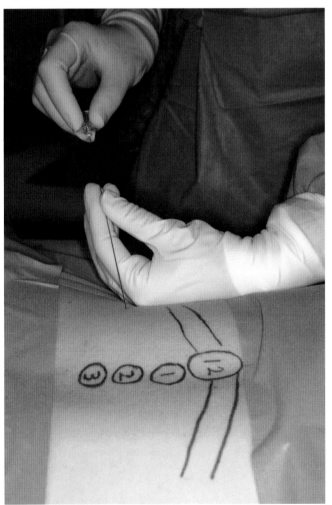

Fig. 5.3.5

- Neurolysis may be achieved by leaving the needle in place after block has been confirmed and injecting 5 ml phenol 6%. To avoid leaving alcohol in the needle tract, the needle is then cleared with air or local anesthetic 1 ml, and removed. However, because of the very high incidence of genitofemoral neuralgia that can occur post-neurolytic lumbar sympathetic block, the benefit versus risk should be considered carefully.
- Monitors should be left attached and i.v. access left in situ for at least 30 minutes.

Confirmation of a successful block

- Increase in skin temperature on the plantar surface of the foot to about 35 °C; temperature should begin to rise in the foot on the side of the block within 3 minutes of injection of local anesthetic.
- Relief of sympathetically maintained pain in the lower limb.

Tips

- If fluoroscopy is not available ultrasound may aid placement of the needle. A line 10 cm from the midline is drawn parallel to the midline; the lowest rib is identified and a line is drawn along its inferior border.
- The point of intersection of these lines should be lateral to the L2 vertebral body.
- Consideration should be given to performance of the block under CT control if the block is unsuccessful.
- Repeated blocks may bring about gradual improvement in sympathetically maintained pain.
- Immediate physiotherapy after blockade may improve the outcome.

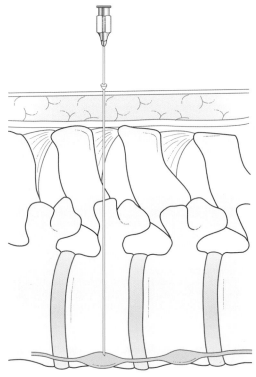

Fig. 5.3.7

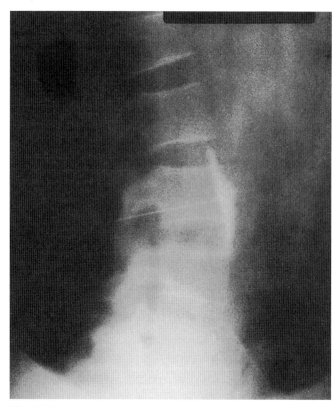

Fig. 5.3.9

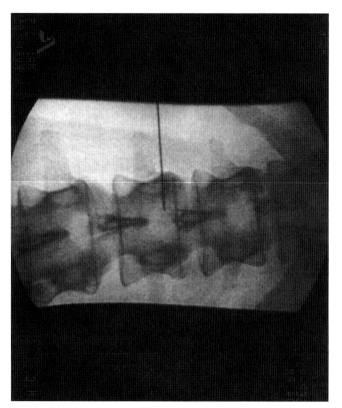

Fig. 5.3.8

Potential problems

- If the needle tip is placed too superficially, the tip may come to lie in the intervertebral foramen and injection may result in a subarachnoid block, an epidural block, or a somatic nerve block. Confirmation of needle position using lateral fluoroscopy is therefore recommended.
- Genitofemoral neuralgia may occur in 5–10% of patients post-neurolytic block causing pain in the groin.
- Perforation of the aorta or the inferior vena cava is possible and retroperitoneal hematoma may occur. Consequently the block should be avoided in patients with coagulopathy.
- Intravascular injection may occur.
- Perforation of the kidney or ureter is usually of no clinical significance unless neurolytic agents are used.
- Perforation of the intervertebral disc may occur. This also is usually of no clinical significance but may produce a septic discitis if bacterial contamination occurs.
- Postural hypotension, secondary to sympathetic blockade, may occur.
- Injection of neurolytic solution into the psoas muscle may cause rhabdomyolysis.
- Patients in the prone position should be monitored carefully when intravenous sedation is administered.

5.4 CELIAC PLEXUS BLOCK—RETROCRURAL APPROACH

Anatomy

The celiac plexus is flat and lies against the crus of the diaphragm, surrounding the root of the celiac and mesenteric arteries and anterior to three vertebral bodies centered at L1. Posteriorly on the left side is the aorta, and on the right is the inferior vena cava. The kidneys lie lateral and the pancreas anterior to the celiac plexus (Fig. 5.4.1 a,b).

The celiac plexus is made up of pre- and postganglionic sympathetic and parasympathetic nerve fibers. Postganglionic sympathetic fibers are supplied from the paired celiac ganglia. Preganglionic sympathetic efferents from the thoracic sympathetic chain are supplied via the greater and lesser splanchnic nerves. The intra-abdominal viscera are supplied by postganglionic sympathetic fibers

that have synapsed in the celiac ganglia (Fig. 5.4.2). The vagus nerve also supplies parasympathetic nerve fibers. Via the celiac plexus dorsal root, ganglion cells innervate the whole of the abdominal viscera, including the liver, spleen, kidneys, suprarenal glands, and intestines, with the exception of the pelvic organs, the rectum, and the left half of the colon.

Pain originating from the viscera is often vague and poorly localized as a result of convergence of neurons in the dorsal horn and crossing over the midline of some of the visceral afferents.

There are two main approaches to celiac plexus blockade. One approach places the two needles posterior to the crura of the diaphragm, the retrocrural approach. The retrocrural approach to the celiac plexus also targets the splanchnic nerves to produce a splanchnic nerve block if required. The other approach places a needle anterior to the crus of the diaphragm on the right, the anterocrural approach (Fig. 5.4.3), as discussed in Section 5.5.

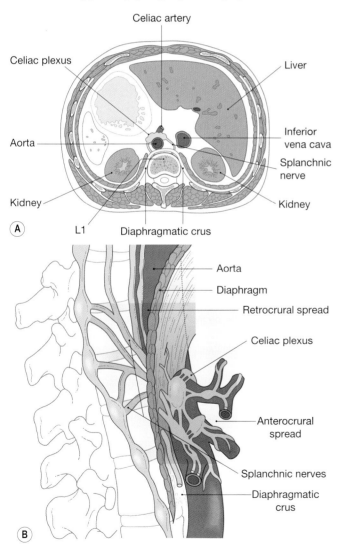

Fig. 5.4.1

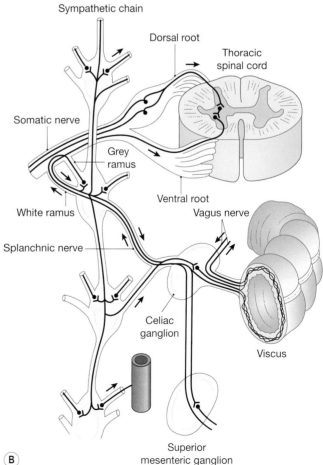

Fig. 5.4.2

Equipment

- 2 ml, 5 ml, and 10 ml syringes
- 30 G needle
- Two 15 cm 22 G needles
- Extension set (optional)
- ECG, BP, SpO$_2$ monitors
- Resuscitation equipment (*see Appendix 3*)
- Fluoroscopy

Drugs

- Mild sedative
- Lidocaine (lignocaine) 1%, 5 ml for skin infiltration
- Lidocaine (lignocaine) 1%, 15–20 ml (or its equivalent) for block
- 6% aqueous phenol or 50–75% alcohol (ethanol). Our suggestion: mix 2 parts absolute alcohol with one part 1% lidocaine. This will help reduce the incidence and severity of pain following injection. In addition, precede all alcohol injections with 3–4 ml 1% lidocaine
- Non-ionic radio-opaque contrast medium
- Resuscitation drugs (*see Appendix 3*)

Position of patient

- Prone.
- Pillow under anterior superior iliac spine to flatten the normal lumbar lordosis (*Fig. 5.4.4*).

Needle puncture and technique

- Intravenous access is inserted.
- Monitors are attached.
- Resuscitation equipment and drugs are checked and made ready for use.
- Mild sedation may be induced.

RETROCRURAL APPROACH

- A 15 cm 22 G spinal needle is selected. A slight curve at the needle tip, away from the bevel direction, may be created, which allows the needle to be redirected during placement.
- An AP view of the upper lumbar/low thoracic spine is obtained and the C-arm is adjusted to superimpose the T12–L1 endplates.
- **A skin wheal is raised at the lower border of the twelfth rib on the right just above the level of the L1 transverse process** (*Fig. 5.4.5 a*). The needle is inserted at this site and advanced at an angle 30° from perpendicular inward until the L1 body is contacted just below the upper endplate (*Fig. 5.4.5*). The curve of the needle is turned laterally and the needle is advanced along the upper portion of the body. Once the needle has slipped a few millimeters past the lateral aspect of the L1 body, a lateral view is obtained. The curve of the needle is directed inward toward the body and advanced until the tip lies at the anterior border of the body, near the upper endplate, in a direct lateral view.
- Using "live" fluoroscopy, 1 ml non-ionic contrast medium is injected. The dye should remain against the anterior aspect of the bodies in the lateral view (*Fig. 5.4.6 a*).
- If dye is seen spreading dorsally toward the neural foramina (*see Fig. 5.4.6 b*), the needle should be withdrawn and repositioned at a higher level.
- An AP view is obtained, which should demonstrate dye spread against the lateral aspect of the bodies (*Fig. 5.4.6 c*).
- Spread more laterally indicates injection within the psoas muscle, in which case the needle should be repositioned more medially and anteriorly. 3 ml 1% lidocaine is then injected. The dye shadow will

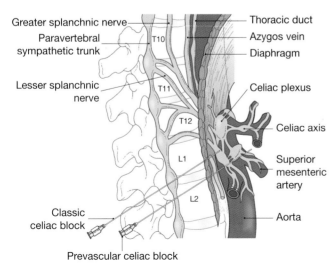

Fig. 5.4.3

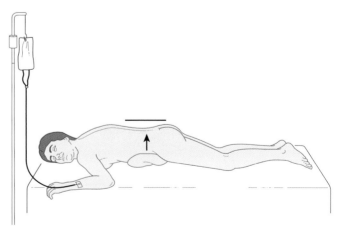

Fig. 5.4.4

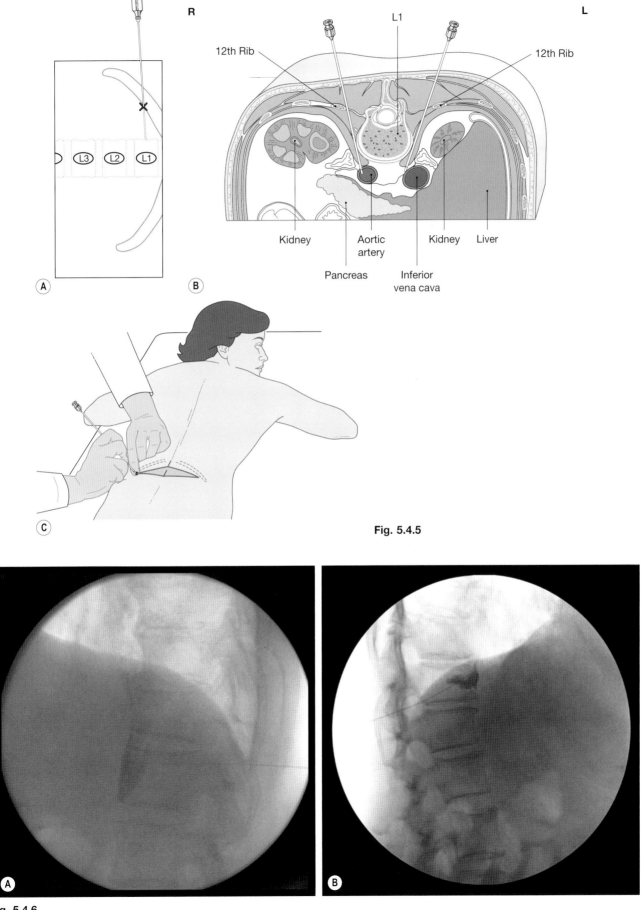

R L

12th Rib L1 12th Rib

Kidney Aortic artery Kidney Liver

Pancreas Inferior vena cava

A B

C

Fig. 5.4.5

A B

Fig. 5.4.6

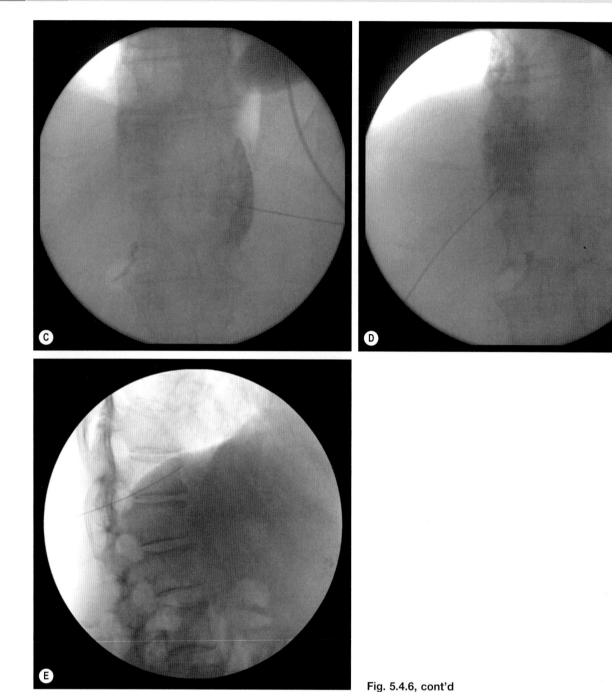

Fig. 5.4.6, cont'd

be seen to expand superiorly, spreading to the thoracic levels to contact the splanchnic nerves (*see Fig. 5.4.6 d*).

- After confirming negative aspiration for blood, 15–20 ml alcohol or phenol is injected. The needle is cleared with 1 ml lidocaine prior to removal.

- Alternatively, the needle can be advanced more cephalad to a position at the anterior border of T12 preferably near either the lower or upper endplate (*Fig. 5.4.6 e*).

- Injection near the mid-point of the body is more likely to result in dorsal spread of the drug toward the neural foramen. More cephalad placement is a bit more difficult technically, but places the needle closer to the splanchnic nerves.

- The procedure is repeated in an identical manner on the left side.

Confirmation of a successful block

- Relief of upper abdominal pain.

Tips

- After injection of non-ionic radio-contrast medium, a blush will indicate injection into muscle. If visible contrast medium disappears immediately it is likely that intravascular injection has occurred.
- Consideration should be given to performance of the block under CT control if the block is unsuccessful.
- Placement of the needle anterior to the diaphragmatic crus can also be achieved via insertion through the abdominal wall.

Potential problems

- The position of each needle tip should always be confirmed with fluoroscopy before injection of neurolytic agent as it may lie in the peritoneal cavity, within a viscus or intravascularly. If a needle tip is placed too superficially, the tip may come to lie in the intervertebral foramen and injection may result in an epidural block or a somatic nerve block. Injection of neurolytic solution into the psoas muscle may cause rhabdomyolysis.
- Perforation of the aorta or the inferior vena cava is possible and consequently the block should be avoided in patients with coagulopathy. Dissection of the aorta may occur as a result of direct damage during the block. Retroperitoneal hematoma may occur and for this reason also the block should be avoided in patients with coagulopathy.
- Orthostatic hypotension may occur as a result of sympathetic blockade for up to 3 days after a neurolytic block. Diarrhea may occur also and hydration of the patient should be monitored.
- Pneumothorax may occur.
- Transient motor paralysis and paraplegia may occur after the block, probably as a result of spasm of the segmental arteries.
- Perforation of the intervertebral disc may occur, but this also is usually of no clinical significance.
- Perforation of the kidney or ureter is usually of no clinical significance unless neurolytic agent is injected.
- The thoracic duct may be damaged (possibly causing chylothorax, or lymphedema).
- Abdominal and chest discomfort may be experienced for 30 minutes after injection of alcohol.
- There may be a detectable odor from the breath after alcohol injection.
- Patients in the prone position should be monitored carefully when intravenous sedation is administered.

5.5 CELIAC PLEXUS BLOCK—ANTEROCRURAL APPROACH

Anatomy

The anterocrural approach places a needle anterior to each crus of the diaphragm. The needles are inserted more medially and directed at a larger angle towards the midline until they come to lie in the retroperitoneal compartment between the aorta, and the inferior vena cava dorsally, and the pancreas ventrally (**Fig. 5.5.1**). Fluoroscopic imaging is necessary for accurate placement of the anterocrural needles using this approach.

Equipment

- 2 ml, 5 ml, and 10 ml syringes
- 30 G needle
- 15 cm 22 G needle (penetration of the diaphragmatic crus is easier with a large gauge needle)
- Extension set (optional)
- ECG, BP, SpO_2 monitors
- Resuscitation equipment (*see Appendix 3*)
- Fluoroscopy

Drugs

- Mild sedative
- Lidocaine (lignocaine) 1%, 5 ml for skin infiltration
- Lidocaine (lignocaine) 1%, 15–20 ml (or its equivalent) for block
- 6% aqueous phenol or 50–75% alcohol (ethanol). Our suggestion: mix 2 parts absolute alcohol with one part 1% lidocaine. This will help reduce the incidence and severity of pain following injection. In addition, precede all alcohol injections with 3–4 ml 1% lidocaine
- Non-ionic radio-opaque contrast medium
- Resuscitation drugs (*see Appendix 3*)

Position of patient

- Prone.
- Pillow under anterior superior iliac spine to flatten the normal lumbar lordosis (*Fig. 5.5.2*).

Needle puncture and technique

- Intravenous access is inserted.
- Monitors are attached.
- Resuscitation equipment and drugs are checked and made ready for use.
- Mild sedation may be induced.

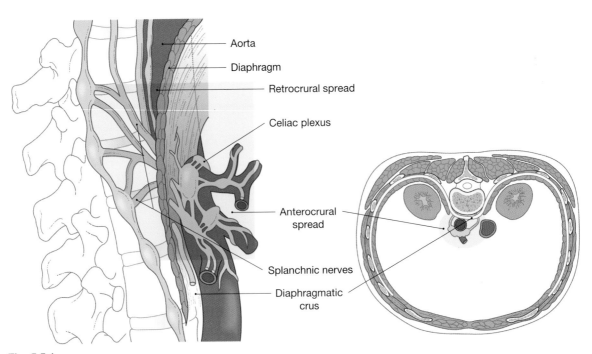

Aorta
Diaphragm
Retrocrural spread
Celiac plexus
Anterocrural spread
Splanchnic nerves
Diaphragmatic crus

Fig. 5.5.1

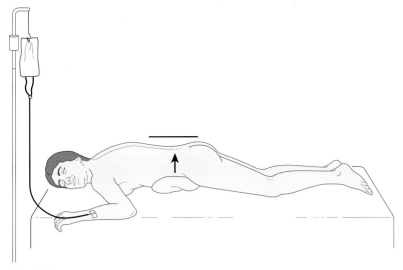

Fig. 5.5.2

- The thoracolumbar midline and area 10 cm × 5 cm laterally is cleaned with antiseptic solution and a fenestrated drape is placed over the sterile area.
- The twelfth rib and L1 are identified and confirmed with fluoroscopy.

ANTEROCRURAL APPROACH

Right side

- A 15 cm 22 G spinal needle is selected. A slight curve at the needle tip, away from the bevel direction, may be created which allows the needle to be redirected during placement.
- An AP view of the upper lumbar/low thoracic spine is obtained and the C-arm is adjusted to superimpose the T12–L1 endplates.
- **A skin wheal is raised at the lower border of the twelfth rib on the right just above the level of the L1 transverse process. The needle is inserted at this site and advanced at an angle 30° from perpendicular inward until the L1 body is contacted just below the upper endplate.**
- The curve of the needle is turned laterally and the needle is advanced along the upper portion of the body.
- Once the needle has slipped a few millimeters past the lateral aspect of the L1 body, a lateral view is obtained.
- The needle is advanced until the tip is 1.5–2 cm anterior to the anterior border of the L1 body. The needle is aspirated and if negative, 1 ml non-ionic contrast is injected. Dye spread should be in an amorphous pattern (*Fig. 5.5.3*).
- If aspiration is negative, 3 ml 1% lidocaine (lignocaine) is injected. If no nerve block is noted after 10 minutes, this is followed by 15–20 ml alcohol. If phenol is used, the lidocaine is not needed.

- 1 ml 1% lidocaine is injected before removing the needle to clear it.

Left side

- **The same procedure is repeated on the left.**
- The needle is positioned 1.5–2 cm anterior to the anterior border of the L1 body. It is then usually within the aorta, and aspiration is positive for arterial blood.
- The needle is advanced forward until aspiration is negative for blood (*Fig. 5.5.3 b*).
- 1 ml contrast is injected. The pattern is generally amorphous anteriorly, but a straight border of dye along the anterior surface of the aorta may be seen (*Fig. 5.4.4*).
- Aspiration is repeated and, if negative, 3 ml 1% lidocaine (lignocaine) is injected. If no nerve block is noted after 10 minutes, this is followed by 15–20 ml alcohol. If phenol is used, the lidocaine is not needed.
- 1 ml 1% lidocaine is injected before removing the needle to clear it.
- Monitors should be left attached and i.v. access left in situ for at least 30 minutes.

Confirmation of a successful block

- Relief of upper abdominal pain.

Tips

- After injection of non-ionic radio-contrast medium, a blush will indicate injection into muscle. If visible contrast medium disappears immediately it is likely that intravascular injection has occurred.
- Consideration should be given to performance of the block under CT control if the block is unsuccessful.

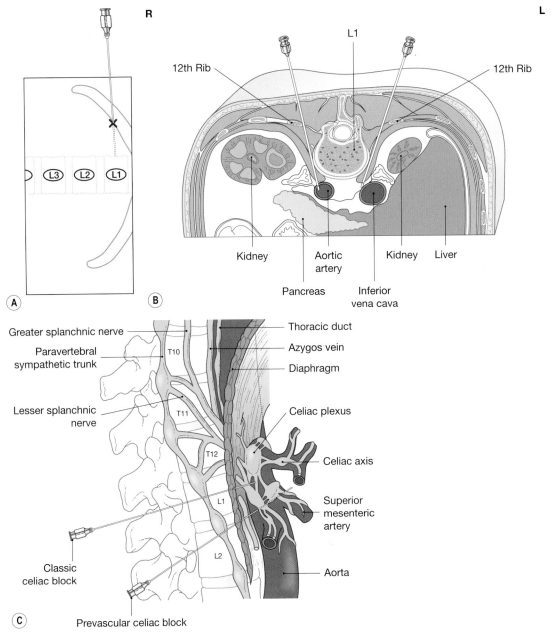

R   L

L1

12th Rib   12th Rib

Kidney   Aortic artery   Kidney   Liver

Pancreas   Inferior vena cava

A   B

Greater splanchnic nerve   Thoracic duct

Paravertebral sympathetic trunk   T10   Azygos vein

Diaphragm

Lesser splanchnic nerve   T11   Celiac plexus

T12   Celiac axis

L1   Superior mesenteric artery

L2   Aorta

Classic celiac block

C

Prevascular celiac block

Fig. 5.5.3

Potential problems

- The position of each needle tip should always be confirmed with fluoroscopy prior to injection of neurolytic agent as it may lie in the peritoneal cavity, within a viscus or intravascularly. If a needle tip is placed too superficially, the tip may come to lie in the intervertebral foramen and injection may result in epidural block or a somatic nerve block. Injection of neurolytic solution into the psoas muscle may cause rhabdomyolysis.

- Perforation of the aorta or the inferior vena cava is possible and consequently the block should be avoided in patients with coagulopathy. Dissection of the aorta may occur as a result of direct damage during the block. Retroperitoneal hematoma may occur and for this reason also the block should be avoided in patients with coagulopathy.

- Orthostatic hypotension may occur as a result of sympathetic blockade for up to three days after a neurolytic block. Diarrhea may occur also and hydration of the patient should be monitored.

- Pneumothorax may occur.
- Transient motor paralysis and paraplegia may occur after the block, probably as a result of spasm of segmental arteries.
- Perforation of the intervertebral disc may occur, but this also is usually of no clinical significance.
- Perforation of the kidney or ureter is usually of no clinical significance unless neurolytic agents are injected.

- The thoracic duct may be damaged (possibly causing chylothorax, or lymphedema).
- Abdominal and chest discomfort may be experienced for 30 minutes after injection of alcohol.
- There may be a detectable odor from the breath after alcohol injection.
- Patients in the prone position should be monitored carefully when intravenous sedation is administered.

5.6 HYPOGASTRIC PLEXUS BLOCK

Anatomy

The superior hypogastric plexus is formed from pelvic sympathetic fibers of the aortic plexus and L2 and L3 splanchnic nerves. These afferent and efferent fibers innervate the pelvic viscera, including the uterus, bladder, vagina, and prostate. The plexus is located between the upper third of the first sacral vertebral body and the lower third of the fifth lumbar vertebral body, at the sacral promontory, in the retroperitoneal space (Fig. 5.6.1 a,b). Parasympathetic nerve fibers from S2–S4 pass through the inferior hypogastric plexus.

Equipment

- 2 ml, 5 ml, and 10 ml syringes
- 30 G needle
- Two 15 cm 22 G needles
- Extension set (optional)
- ECG, BP, and SpO₂ monitors
- Resuscitation equipment (*see Appendix 3*)
- Fluoroscopy

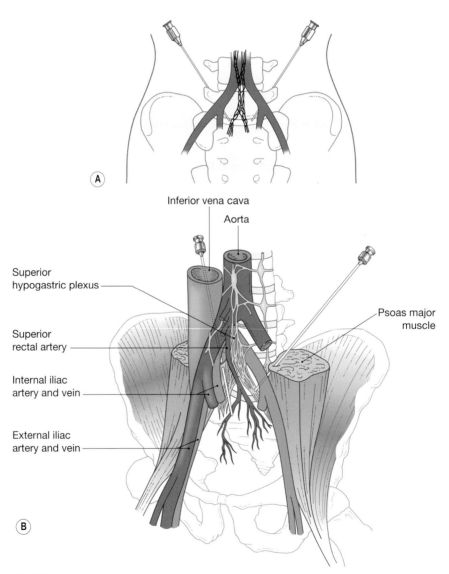

(A)

Inferior vena cava

Aorta

Superior hypogastric plexus

Superior rectal artery

Internal iliac artery and vein

External iliac artery and vein

Psoas major muscle

(B)

Fig. 5.6.1

Drugs

- Lidocaine (lignocaine) 1%, 5 ml for skin infiltration
- Lidocaine (lignocaine) 1%, 15–20 ml (or its equivalent) for block
- Phenol 6%
- Non-ionic radio-opaque contrast medium
- Resuscitation drugs (*see Appendix 3*)

Position of patient

- Prone.
- Pillow under anterior superior iliac spine to flatten the normal lumbar lordosis (*Fig. 5.6.2*).

Needle puncture and technique

- Intravenous access is inserted.
- Monitors are attached.
- Resuscitation equipment and drugs are checked and made ready for use.
- The lumbosacral midline and area 10 cm × 5 cm laterally is cleaned with antiseptic solution and a fenestrated drape is placed over the sterile area.
- The iliac crests are palpated and the intercrestal line is identified (this corresponds with the inferior aspect of the spinous process of L4 or may lie in the L4–5 interspace).
- The spinous processes are counted until the L5–S1 interspace is identified and confirmed with fluoroscopy.
- **The insertion points lie 2 cm lateral and 2 cm cephalad to the space between the L5 transverse process and the sacrum** (*Fig. 5.6.3 a,b*).
- A skin wheal is raised at one of the marked sites and the area is infiltrated with lidocaine (lignocaine) 1%.
- At a 30° angle to the frontal plane, a 22 G 15 cm needle is advanced, aimed slightly caudad towards the L5–S1 interspace (*Fig. 5.6.3 c*), until the lower part of

the L5 vertebral body is contacted at a depth of about 7–9 cm and confirmed with fluoroscopy. If the needle contacts bone at a more superficial level, it is probable that it has come into contact with the L5 transverse process or the sacrum and needs to be repositioned.
- The needle depth is noted.
- The needle is then withdrawn to the subcutaneous tissue and, with the aid of fluoroscopy, it is re-advanced, this time at an angle 45° to the frontal plane (or with slight concavity of the needle) until the previous depth (as noted) is reached. It should slip past the vertebral body at a depth about 1–2 cm deeper than the first depth mark, to lie just anterior to the upper portion of the sacrum (*Fig. 5.6.4*).
- After negative aspiration, the fluoroscopic image is observed as a small amount of non-ionic radio-contrast medium is injected (*Fig. 5.6.5*). The correct placement of the needle is indicated by the presence of a collection of contrast medium just anterior to the upper portion of the sacrum or the L5–S1 interspace (*Fig. 5.6.6*). The contrast medium usually spreads in all directions, not usually along the sacrum.
- The procedure is repeated on the other side in a mirrored fashion (*Figs 5.6.7, 5.6.8*).
- After further negative aspirations, 5 ml of lidocaine (lignocaine) 1% is injected bilaterally and the patient is questioned about pain relief. There should be little resistance to injection, similar to that felt when injecting through an epidural needle. If resistance is encountered, or if the injection is painful, the needle should be repositioned.
- After 10 minutes the patient is questioned about pain relief and any symptoms of somatic nerve blockade. Sensory and motor functioning of the lower extremities is checked. The procedure should be abandoned if there is evidence of somatic blockade.
- After confirmation of pain relief and lack of somatic block, 6 ml phenol 6% is injected through each needle using glass syringes. The needles are then cleared with air or local anesthetic 1 ml, and removed.
- Monitors should be left attached and i.v. access left in situ for at least 30 minutes.
- Ultrasound may help placement of the needle (*Figs 5.6.9–5.6.10*).

Confirmation of a successful block

- Relief of lower abdominal pain.

Tips

- After injection of non-ionic radio-contrast medium, a blush will indicate injection into muscle. If this disappears immediately it is likely that intravascular injection has occurred.

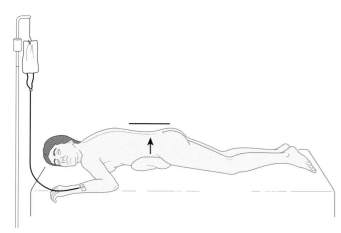

Fig. 5.6.2

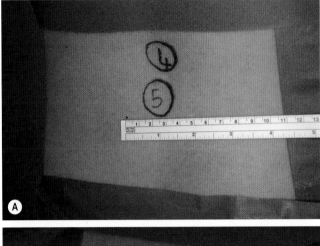

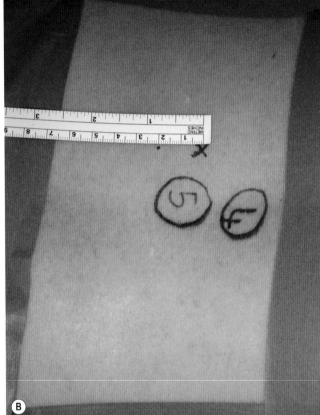

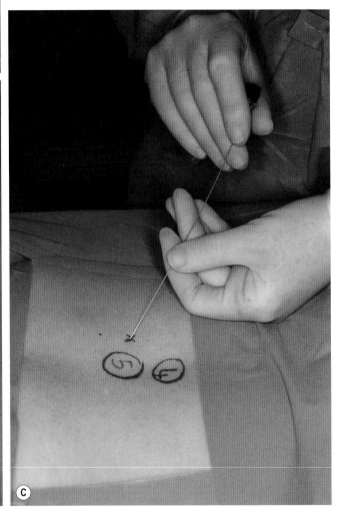

Fig. 5.6.3

• Consideration should be given to performance of the block under CT control if the block is unsuccessful (*Fig. 5.6.10*).

Potential problems

• The position of each needle tip should always be confirmed with fluoroscopy prior to injection of neurolytic agents as it may lie in the peritoneal cavity, within a viscus or intravascularly. If a needle tip is placed too superficially, the tip may come to lie in the intervertebral foramen and injection may result in an epidural block or a somatic nerve block. Injection of neurolytic solution into the psoas muscle may cause rhabdomyolysis.

• Perforation of the aorta or the inferior vena cava is possible and consequently the block should be avoided in patients with coagulopathy. Dissection of the aorta may occur as a result of direct damage during the block. Retroperitoneal hematoma may occur and for this reason also the block should be avoided in patients with coagulopathy.

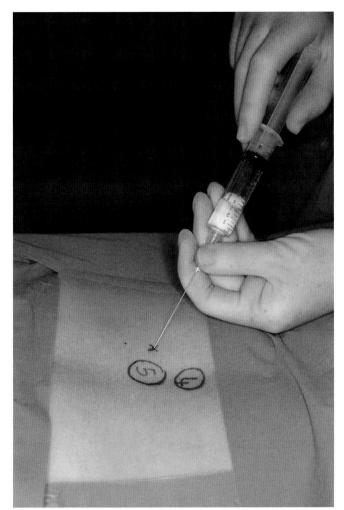

Fig. 5.6.4

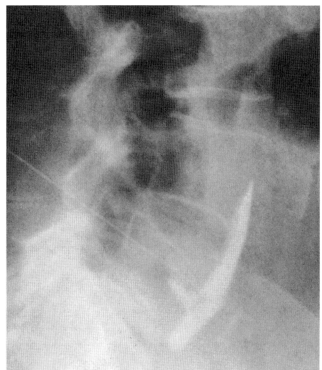

Fig. 5.6.6

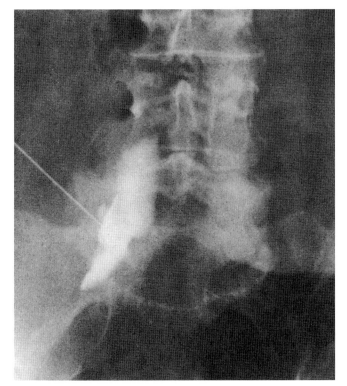

Fig. 5.6.5

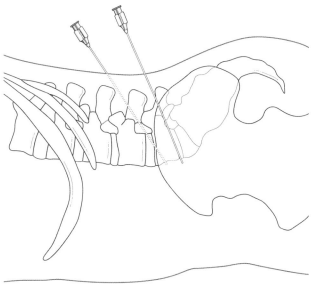

Fig. 5.6.7

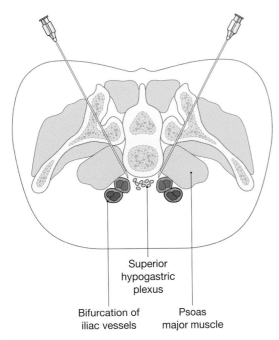

Superior
hypogastric
plexus

Bifurcation of
iliac vessels

Psoas
major muscle

Fig. 5.6.8

- Orthostatic hypotension may occur as a result of sympathetic blockade for up to three days after a neurolytic block. Diarrhea may occur also and hydration of the patient should be monitored.
- Transient motor paralysis and paraplegia may occur after the block, probably as a result of spasm of segmental arteries.
- Perforation of the intervertebral disc may occur, but this is usually of no clinical significance.

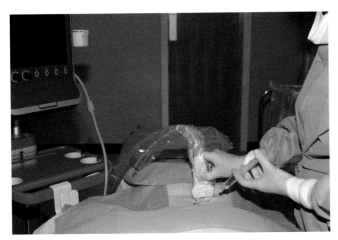

Fig. 5.6.9

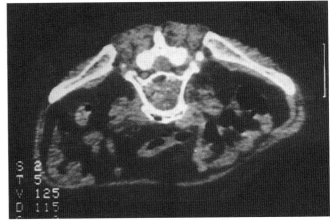

Fig. 5.6.10

5.7 GANGLION IMPAR BLOCK

Anatomy

The ganglion impar is a retroperitoneal sympathetic ganglion located at the level of the sacrococcygeal junction (Fig. 5.7.1). Above the level of this ganglion the sympathetic chains are paired. Sympathetic afferents from the perineum, distal rectum and anus, distal urethra, vulva and the distal third of the vagina converge in the ganglion impar.

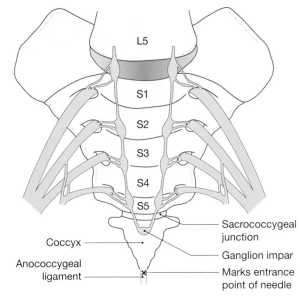

Fig. 5.7.1

Equipment

- 2ml, 5 ml, and 10 ml syringes
- 30 G needle
- 22 G spinal needle
- Extension set (optional)
- ECG, BP, and SpO$_2$ monitors
- Resuscitation equipment (*see Appendix 3*)

Drugs

- Lidocaine (lignocaine) 1%, 5 ml for skin infiltration
- Lidocaine (lignocaine) 1%, 15–20 ml (or its equivalent) for block
- Phenol 6%
- Non-ionic radio-opaque contrast medium
- Resuscitation drugs (*see Appendix 3*)

Position of patient

- Prone.
- Pillow under anterior superior iliac spine to flatten the normal lumbar lordosis (*Fig. 5.7.2*).

Needle puncture and technique

- Intravenous access is inserted.
- Monitors are attached.
- Resuscitation equipment and drugs are checked and made ready for use.
- The midline along the intergluteal groove and an area 10 cm × 5 cm laterally is cleaned with antiseptic

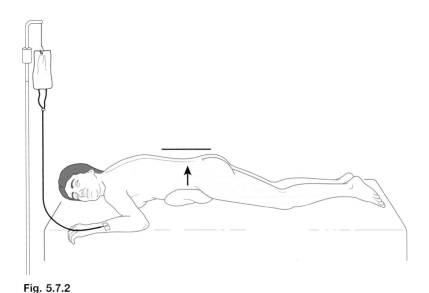

Fig. 5.7.2

solution and a fenestrated drape is placed over the sterile area.

- A skin wheal is raised at the superior aspect of the intergluteal groove, just above the anus, over the anococcygeal ligament (*Fig. 5.7.3*).
- The stylet from the 22 G spinal needle is removed, and the needle is bent with the fingers to form a 30° angle, approximately 2 cm from the hub.
- The needle is inserted through the skin wheal, with the concave curvature facing posteriorly.
- With the aid of fluoroscopy, the needle is advanced deep into the coccyx, closely approximating its anterior surface, until the tip reaches the level of the sacrococcygeal junction (*Fig. 5.7.4*).

- After negative aspiration, the fluoroscopic image is observed as a small amount of non-ionic radio-contrast medium is injected. The correct placement of the needle is indicated by the presence a small round blob of contrast medium at the anterior border of the vertebral column (*Fig. 5.7.5 a,b*).
- Lidocaine (lignocaine) 1% 5 ml is injected for ganglion blockade.

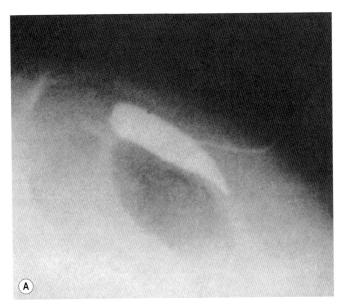

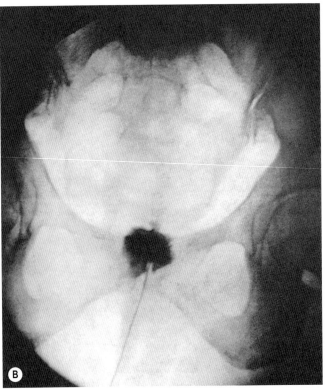

Fig. 5.7.5

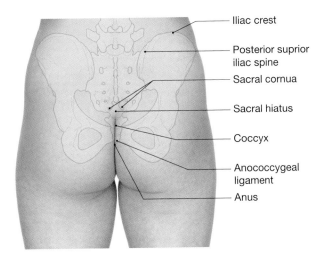

Fig. 5.7.3

- Iliac crest
- Posterior suprior iliac spine
- Sacral cornua
- Sacral hiatus
- Coccyx
- Anococcygeal ligament
- Anus

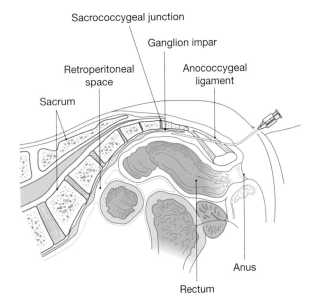

Sacrococcygeal junction
Ganglion impar
Retroperitoneal space
Anococcygeal ligament
Sacrum
Anus
Rectum

Fig. 5.7.4

- After 10 minutes the patient is questioned about pain relief and any somatic blockade. Sensory and motor functioning of the lower extremities is checked. The procedure should be abandoned if there is evidence of somatic blockade.
- After confirmation of pain relief and lack of somatic block, 5 ml of phenol 6% is injected using a glass syringe. To avoid leaving alcohol in the needle tract the needle is then cleared with air or local anesthetic 1 ml, and removed.
- Monitors should be left attached and i.v. access left in situ for at least 30 minutes.

Confirmation of a successful block

- Relief of perineal pain.

Tips

- To aid access to the anococcygeal ligament an assistant may be asked to retract the skin of the buttock; after penetration of the skin, this is no longer required.
- Exaggerated anterior curvature of the sacrococcygeal vertebral column may inhibit access and it may be necessary to bend the needle to a more acute angle.

Potential problems

- The position of each needle tip should always be confirmed with fluoroscopy prior to injection of neurolytic agent as it may lie in the peritoneal cavity, within a viscus or intravascularly. Caudal epidural placement of the needle is possible, therefore it is essential that spread of contrast material is observed to be restricted to the retroperitoneum, and that a test dose produces no somatic nerve blockade. Perforation of the rectum or periosteal injection is also possible.
- Local tumor invasion may inhibit spread of solution.
- Retroperitoneal hematoma may occur and the block should be avoided in patients with coagulopathy. Diarrhea may occur also and hydration of the patient should be monitored.
- There may be a detectable odor from the breath after alcohol injection.
- Patients in the prone position should be monitored carefully when intravenous sedation is administered.

5.8 INTRAVENOUS REGIONAL SYMPATHETIC BLOCK—UPPER LIMB

Anatomy

Peripheral sympathetic blockade is achieved by limiting the effect of the sympatholytic agent to the tissues of the affected limb using a tourniquet. Intravenous injection of an agent that releases endogenous norepinephrine (noradrenaline) from sympathetic nerve endings causes depletion of this neurotransmitter, and thereby chemical sympathetic blockade.

Equipment

- 20 ml syringe
- Two i.v. cannulae
- Pneumatic tourniquet
- ECG, BP, and SpO$_2$ monitors
- Skin temperature monitor
- Resuscitation equipment (*see Appendix 3*)

Drugs

- Lidocaine (lignocaine) 0.5% *without epinephrine/adrenaline*, or its equivalent
- Bretylium 1.5 mg/kg (or its equivalent, e.g. guanethedine 0.25 mg/kg)
- Saline (NaCl) 20 ml
- Resuscitation drugs (*see Appendix 3*)

Position of patient

- Supine.

Technique

- Intravenous access is inserted in the contralateral limb.
- Peripheral i.v. access is inserted in the limb to be blocked (*Fig. 5.8.1 a*).
- Monitors are attached.

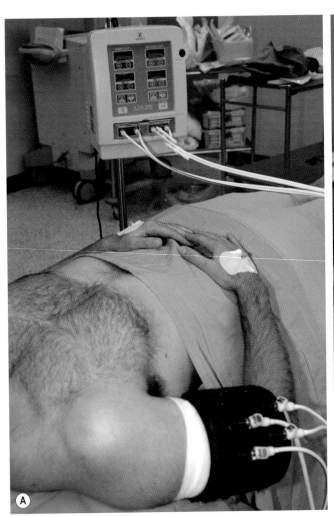

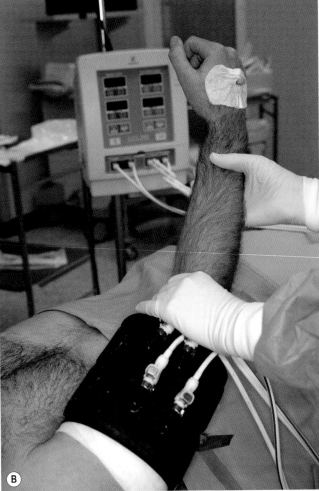

Fig. 5.8.1

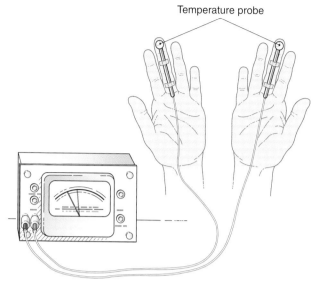
Temperature probe

Fig. 5.8.3

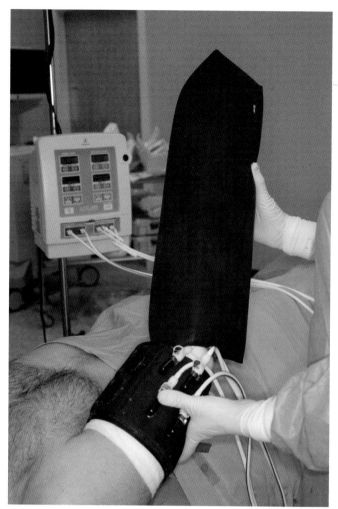

Fig. 5.8.2

- Resuscitation equipment and drugs are checked and made ready for use.
- The limb is raised above the level of the heart for 2 minutes (*Fig. 5.8.1 b*).
- With the limb raised, it is exsanguinated by applying a tight wrap, e.g. Esmarch bandage.
- A thin layer of padding is applied, e.g. Velband, under the tourniquet site.
- The tourniquet is applied and the cuff is inflated to a pressure 100 mmHg higher than the systolic blood pressure (*Fig. 5.8.2*).
- The limb is then lowered. A mixture of lidocaine (lignocaine) 0.5% 15 ml (*without epinephrine/adrenaline*), bretylium 1.5 mg/kg (or guanethidine 0.25 mg/kg), and NaCl to make a total volume of 40 ml (a final lidocaine (lignocaine) solution of 0.25%), is injected through the i.v. cannula in the affected limb.
- The tourniquet is allowed to remain inflated for at least 30 minutes.

- It is then deflated in one step, but left in place. Re-inflation may be required if there is a precipitous change in blood pressure.
- Monitors should be left attached and i.v. access left in situ for at least 30 minutes.

Confirmation of a successful block

- Relief of sympathetically maintained pain.
- Measurements of skin temperature of the affected limb before and after the block should demonstrate temperature increase. However, the sympatholytic effect of the drug may not be immediate (*Fig. 5.8.3*).

Tips

- If i.v. access to the affected limb is difficult due to vasoconstriction, a smear of glycerol trinitrate cream on the dorsum of the hand will usually aid i.v. insertion.
- A single or double cuff may be employed for this block but a double tourniquet may make the block more comfortable. The proximal cuff is inflated first. A few minutes after injection the distal cuff is inflated and **when inflation is complete the proximal cuff is released**.
- Retrograde cannulation, i.e. towards the periphery (*Figs 5.8.4, 5.8.5*) rather than proximally (*Figs 5.8.6, 5.8.7*), may help direct the spread of bretylium to the periphery.
- Active or passive movements of the limb may hasten the distribution of bretylium to the periphery.
- If the tourniquet inflation is painful, inhalation of nitrous oxide–oxygen mixture may improve comfort.
- Repeated blocks may bring about gradual improvement in sympathetically maintained pain.

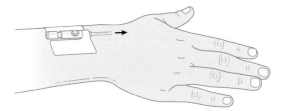

Fig. 5.8.4

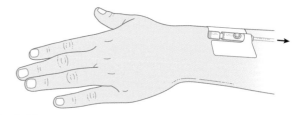

Fig. 5.8.6

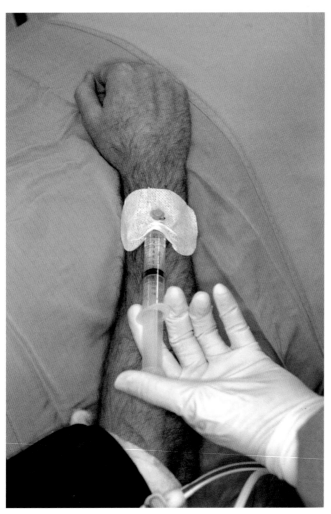

Fig. 5.8.5

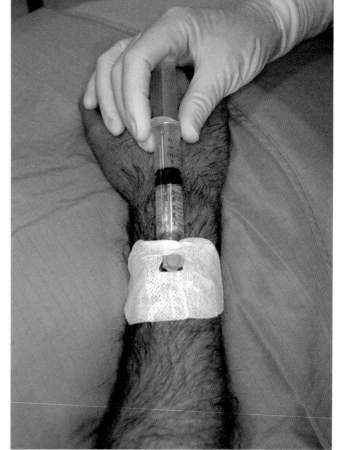

Fig. 5.8.7

- Immediate physiotherapy after block may improve outcome.

Potential problems

- Accidental deflation of the tourniquet early in the procedure may cause a precipitous rise in blood pressure due to the general release of endogenous norepinephrine/noradrenaline when unfixed bretylium enters the circulation. Systemic toxicity of lidocaine (lignocaine) may also occur, possibly causing seizures. Blood pressure may decrease after deflation of the cuff later in the procedure.
- The tourniquet inflation may be painful.
- A sensation of burning may occur after injection due to release of endogenous norepinephrine.
- Neuropraxia may occur (rarely) with a very tight tourniquet.
- Avoid in sickle cell anemia.

5.9 INTRAVENOUS REGIONAL SYMPATHETIC BLOCK—LOWER LIMB

Anatomy

As in the case of the upper limb, peripheral sympathetic blockade is achieved by limiting the effect of the sympatholytic agent to the tissues of the affected limb using a tourniquet. Intravenous injection of an agent releases endogenous norepinephrine (noradrenaline) from sympathetic nerve endings, which causes depletion of this neurotransmitter, and may bring about a chemical sympathetic block.

Equipment

- 50 ml syringe
- Two i.v. cannulae
- Pneumatic tourniquet
- ECG, BP, and SpO$_2$ monitors
- Skin temperature monitor
- Resuscitation equipment (*see Appendix 3*)

Drugs

- Lidocaine (lignocaine) 0.5% *without epinephrine (adrenaline)*, or its equivalent
- Bretylium 1.5 mg/kg (or its equivalent, e.g. guanethedine 0.5 mg/kg)
- Saline (NaCl) 30 ml
- Resuscitation drugs (*see Appendix 3*)

Position of patient

- Supine.

Technique

- Intravenous access is inserted in the contralateral limb.
- Peripheral i.v. access is inserted in the limb to be blocked.
- Monitors are attached.
- Resuscitation equipment and drugs are checked and made ready for use.
- The limb is raised above the level of the heart for 2 minutes (*Fig. 5.9.1*).
- With the limb raised, it is exsanguinated by applying a tight wrap (*Fig. 5.9.2*).
- A thin layer of padding is applied, e.g. Velband, under the tourniquet site.
- The tourniquet is applied and inflated to a pressure 100 mmHg higher than the systolic blood pressure. A second tourniquet may be applied to the calf of patients with no known predispositions to deep venous thrombosis. Inflation of this second cuff may aid limitation of spread of sympatholytic agent to the periphery (*Fig. 5.9.3*).
- The limb is then lowered and a mixture of lidocaine (lignocaine) 0.5% 25 ml (*without epinephrine*), bretylium 1.5 mg/kg (or its equivalent) and NaCl to make a total volume of 40 ml (a final lidocaine/lignocaine solution of 0.25%) is injected through the i.v. cannula in the affected limb.
- The tourniquet is allowed to remain inflated for at least 30 minutes.
- It is then deflated in one step, but left in place. Re-inflation may be required if there is a precipitous change in blood pressure.

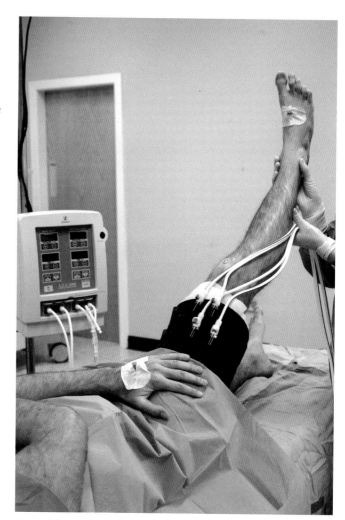

Fig. 5.9.1

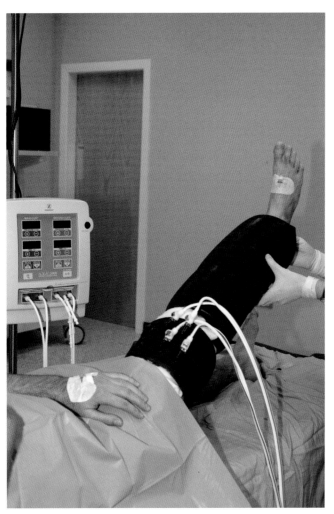

Fig. 5.9.2

- Monitors should be left attached and i.v. access left in situ for at least 30 minutes.

Confirmation of a successful block

- Relief of sympathetically maintained pain.
- Measurements of skin temperature of the affected limb before and after the block should demonstrate temperature increase (*Fig. 5.9.4*).

Tips

- If i.v. access to the affected limb is difficult due to vasoconstriction, a smear of glycerol trinitrate cream on the dorsum of the foot will usually aid i.v. insertion.
- A single or double cuff may be employed for this block but a double tourniquet may make the block more comfortable. The proximal cuff is inflated first. A few minutes after injection the distal cuff is inflated and when inflation is complete the proximal cuff is released.
- Retrograde cannulation, i.e. towards the periphery (*Fig. 5.9.5*) rather than proximally (*see Fig. 5.9.3*), may help direct the spread of bretylium to the periphery.
- Active or passive movements of the limb may hasten the distribution of bretylium to the periphery.
- If the tourniquet inflation is painful, inhalation of nitrous oxide–oxygen mixture may improve comfort.
- Repeated blocks may bring about gradual improvement in sympathetically maintained pain.
- Immediate physiotherapy after block may improve outcome.

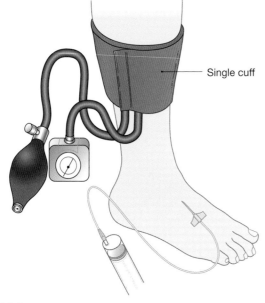

Single cuff

Fig. 5.9.3

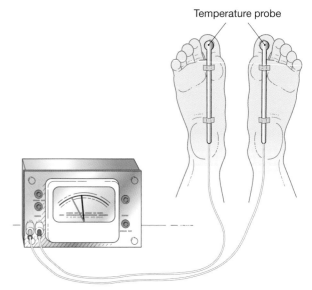

Temperature probe

Fig. 5.9.4

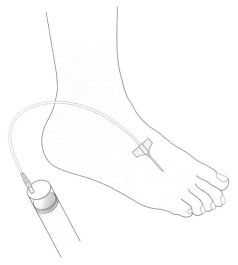

Fig. 5.9.5

Potential problems

- Accidental deflation of the tourniquet early in the procedure may cause a precipitous rise in blood pressure due to the general release of endogenous norepinephrine or epinephrine when unfixed bretylium enters the circulation. Systemic toxicity of lidocaine (lignocaine) may also occur in high doses possibly causing seizures. Blood pressure may decrease after deflation of the cuff later in the procedure.
- The tourniquet inflation may be painful.
- A sensation of burning may occur after injection due to release of endogenous norepinephrine.
- Neuropraxia may occur (rarely) with a very tight tourniquet.
- Avoid in sickle cell anemia.

MUSCLE INJECTIONS 6

Myofascial pain occurs commonly in the muscles of the upper and lower back. It is characterized by pain associated with movement of the affected muscles that develop areas of extreme tenderness, termed trigger points. Palpation of these points is usually perceived as a tight band or firm nodule in the muscle and reproduces pain that may be referred some distance from the site of palpation. Involuntary muscular contraction can occur on palpation, and snapping palpation can result in a local twitch response. Electromyography (EMG) is not reliable in diagnosing myofascial pain syndrome and it is worth remembering that this syndrome may occur in association with underlying painful disorders of the spine.

Injection of trigger points with local anesthetic, especially if repeated several times and combined with stretching exercises, may have a beneficial therapeutic effect on the pain of myofascial pain syndrome. Pain reproduction during injection, followed by relief of pain after injection, that lasts at least as long as the expected local anesthetic effect, indicates that these painful points contribute to myofascial pain syndrome.

Fibromyalgia is a pain syndrome characterized by widespread, diffuse and usually symmetrical tender areas of muscles. Bony structures, such as costochondral junctions and lateral epicondyles, produce local pain, but not referred, on palpation of tender points. Injection of these tender areas typically does not improve the pain of fibromyalgia.

Usually a dilute solution of local anesthetic suffices for beneficial effect. Bupivacaine produces more muscle degeneration than any other local anesthetic when injected into a muscle, and consequently it is usually avoided, lidocaine (lignocaine) being the usual local anesthetic of choice.

The optimum number of trigger-point injections required to produce pain relief is variable. The injection sites may themselves be painful after the local anesthetic wears off. This may exacerbate muscle spasm if too many trigger-point injections are performed. Consideration should be given to the severity of the muscle spasm, the number of trigger points, and to the sensitivity of the patient to pain when deciding on the number of injections.

6.1 TRIGGER-POINT INJECTIONS—NECK AND THORAX

Anatomy

The muscles most often involved in myofascial pain syndrome of the neck include the trapezius, rhomboid minor and major, latissimus dorsi, levator scapulae and splenius capitis (Fig. 6.1.1; see also Fig. 2.1.2).

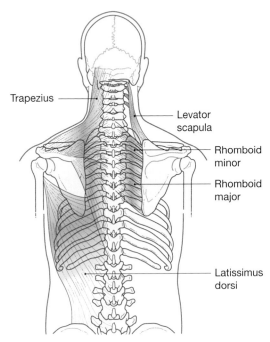

Fig. 6.1.1

Trapezius
Levator scapula
Rhomboid minor
Rhomboid major
Latissimus dorsi

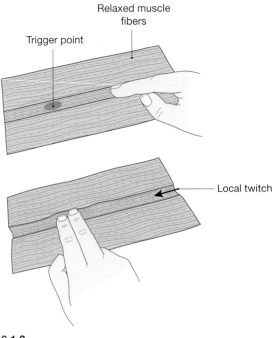

Relaxed muscle fibers
Trigger point
Local twitch

Fig. 6.1.2

Equipment

- 10 ml syringe
- 25 G needle

Drugs

- Lidocaine (lignocaine) 1% 10 ml

Position of patient

- Prone.
- Pillow under chest to allow the neck to flex.
- The sitting position is also used, but vasovagal response may follow trigger-point injections especially in young adults, and it is probably more prudent to use the prone position.

Needle puncture and technique

- The neck, shoulders, and upper posterior thorax are cleaned with antiseptic solution.
- **Trigger points in the muscles are palpated (Fig. 6.1.2) and marked** (*Fig. 6.1.3*).
- A 25 G needle with syringe attached is inserted into a trigger point (*Fig. 6.1.4*).
- After negative aspiration, 2–3 ml of lidocaine (lignocaine) 1% is injected into the trigger point while moving the needle back and forth through the muscle.
- After injection, the next trigger point is injected in the same manner (*Fig. 6.1.5 a,b*).

Confirmation of a successful injection

- Pain reproduction when the needle enters the muscle confirms correct placement.

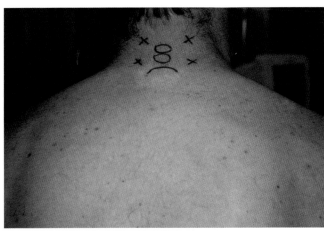

Fig. 6.1.3

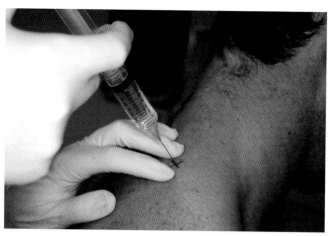

Fig. 6.1.4

Tips

- For best results, injection is carried out in a fan-like manner by repeatedly withdrawing the needle slightly and redirecting it.
- Stretching of the involved muscles by physiotherapy within the duration of the local anesthesia improves results.
- Some workers advocate massage of the area immediately after injection.

Potential problems

- Pain on injection.
- Vasovagal response (especially in young adults in the sitting position).
- Pneumothorax (especially in thin patients).

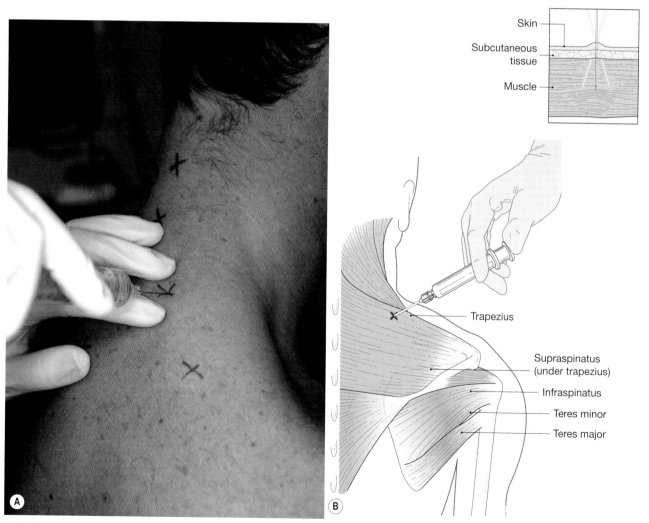

Fig. 6.1.5

6.2 TRIGGER-POINT INJECTIONS—BACK

Anatomy

The muscles most often involved in myofascial pain syndrome of the back include the erector spinae (the longissimus, iliocostalis, and spinalis columns) and the deep transversospinal (semispinalis, multifidus, and rotatores) muscles (Fig. 6.2.1 a,b). In the buttocks, spasm of the gluteus medius muscle may also cause significant pain.

Equipment

- 10 ml syringe
- 25 G needle

Drugs

- Lidocaine (lignocaine) 1% 10 ml

Position of patient

- Prone.
- Pillow under abdomen to straighten the normal lumbar lordosis (Fig. 6.2.2 a).
- The sitting position is also used, but vasovagal response may follow trigger-point injections, and it is probably more prudent to use the prone position.
- Alternatively, the semiprone position will also allow access to affected muscles (Fig. 6.2.2 b).

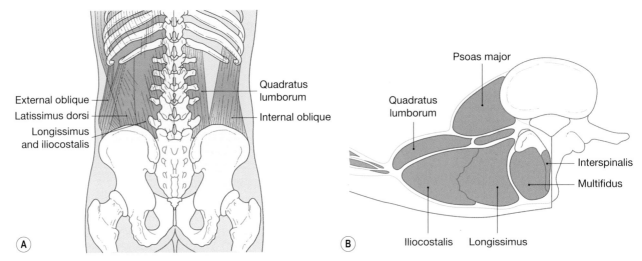

Fig. 6.2.1

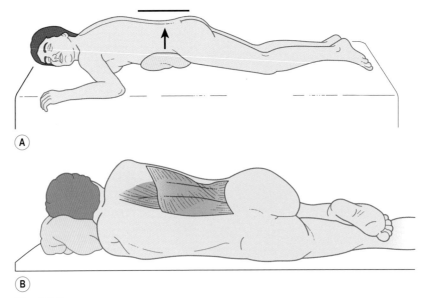

Fig. 6.2.2

Needle puncture and technique

- The midline and the surrounding area are cleaned with antiseptic solution.
- **Trigger points in the muscles are identified by palpation and marked** (*Fig. 6.2.3*).
- A 25 G needle with syringe attached is inserted into a trigger point (*Fig. 6.2.4*).
- After negative aspiration, 2–3 ml of lidocaine (lignocaine) 1% is injected into the trigger point while moving the needle back and forth through the muscle (*Fig. 6.2.5*).

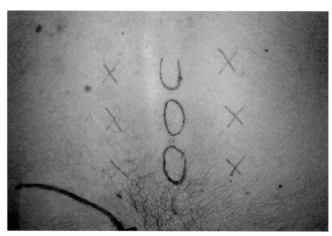

Fig. 6.2.3

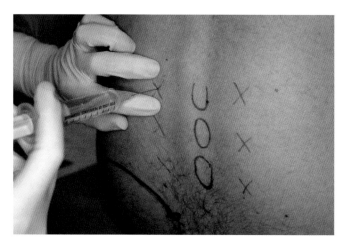

Fig. 6.2.4

- After injection, the next trigger point is injected in the same manner.

Confimation of a successful injection

- Pain reproduction when the needle enters the muscle confirms correct placement.

Tips

- For best results, injection is carried out in a fan-like manner by repeatedly withdrawing the needle slightly and redirecting it.
- Stretching of the involved muscles by physiotherapy within the duration of the local anesthetic improves results.
- Some workers advocate massage of the area immediately after injection.

Potential problems

- Pain on injection.
- Vasovagal response (especially young adults in the sitting position).
- Pneumothorax (especially in thin patients) is also a possibility when injecting the upper back.

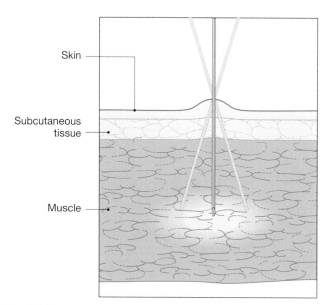

Skin

Subcutaneous tissue

Muscle

Fig. 6.2.5

6.3 GLUTEUS MEDIUS INJECTION

Anatomy

When the buttock muscles are relaxed the quadratus femoris, gemelli and gluteus medius muscles can be palpated. Spasm of the gluteus medius muscle (Fig. 6.3.1) may be the source of buttock pain and may respond to trigger-point injection. Unlike piformis muscle spasm, this does not produce symptoms of sciatic nerve irritation but causes localized pain, often referred to the posterior thigh and calf.

Equipment

- 10 ml syringe
- 22 G needle

Drugs

- Lidocaine (lignocaine) 1% 10 ml

Position of patient

- Prone.
- Pillow under abdomen to flatten the normal lumbar lordosis (Fig. 6.3.2).

Needle puncture and technique

- The surface of the buttock and hip is cleaned with antiseptic solution.
- The posterior superior iliac spine is palpated and marked.
- The greater trochanter is palpated.
- **The insertion point of the needle lies approximately 2 cm medial and superior to the greater trochanter** (Figs 6.3.3, 6.3.4).
- A 22 G needle is introduced in a direction vertical to the skin and advanced until it is felt to be gripped by the tense muscle (Fig. 6.3.5).

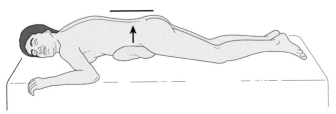

Fig. 6.3.2

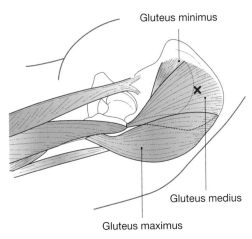

Gluteus minimus

Gluteus medius

Gluteus maximus

Fig. 6.3.3

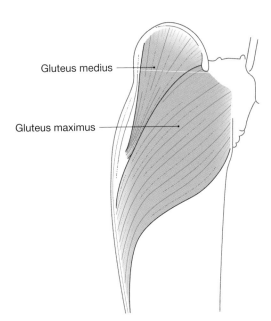

Gluteus medius

Gluteus maximus

Fig. 6.3.1

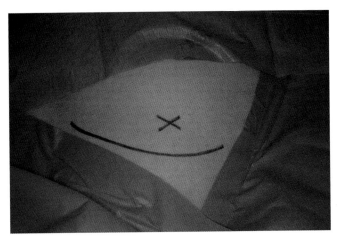

Fig. 6.3.4

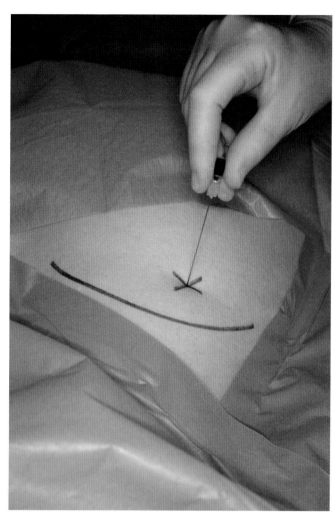

Fig. 6.3.5

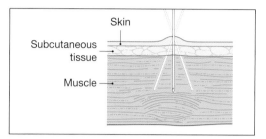

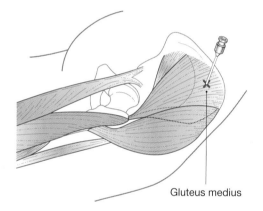

Fig. 6.3.6

- After negative aspiration, lidocaine (lignocaine) 1% 3 ml is injected in the substance of the muscle while moving the needle back and forth in the muscle (*Fig. 6.3.6*).
- The procedure is repeated if other trigger points are present in the muscle.

Confirmation of a successful injection

- Pain reproduction when the needle enters the muscle confirms correct placement of the needle.
- Relief of pain on abduction of the hip.

Tips

- For best results injection is carried out in a fan-like manner by repeatedly withdrawing the needle slightly and redirecting it (*see inset in Fig. 6.3.6*).

Potential problems

- Sciatic nerve block: although this is unusual because the injection site is not very close to the sciatic notch, it is prudent to warn the patient of the possibility.
- Infection or abscess formation.

6.4 PIRIFORMIS INJECTION

Anatomy

The piriformis muscle inserts into the pelvic surface of the sacrum from the second to the fourth segments, lateral to the anterior sacral foramina, and passes out of the pelvis through the greater sciatic foramen to insert into the superior aspect of the greater trochanter (**Fig. 6.4.1**). It overlies the sciatic nerve in the greater sciatic foramen. Contraction contributes to abduction of the lower limb. Spasm of the muscle in myofascial pain syndrome often causes pain referred to the posterior thigh and calf.

Equipment

- 2 ml syringe and two 5 ml syringes
- 25 G needle
- 22 G spinal needle, end-opening

Drugs

- Lidocaine (lignocaine) 1% 10 ml (or its equivalent)

Position of patient

- Prone.
- Pillow under abdomen to flatten the normal lumbar lordosis (*Fig. 6.4.2*).

Needle puncture and technique

- The surface of the buttock and hip is cleaned with antiseptic solution and a fenestrated drape is placed over the sterile area.
- The posterior superior iliac spine is palpated and marked.
- The greater trochanter is palpated and marked.
- **The insertion points of the needle lie at the points one-third and two-thirds along, and 1–3 cm below the line connecting these two marks** (*Figs 6.4.3 a,b,c*).
- The first insertion point, the medial one, is infiltrated with lidocaine (lignocaine) 1% 2 ml.
- A 22 G spinal needle is introduced in a direction vertical to the skin and advanced until it is felt to be gripped by the tense piriformis muscle, or until bone is contacted (*Figs 6.4.4, 6.4.5*).
- The end-point is a fascial click at a depth of about 4–5 cm, depending on the thickness of adipose tissue.
- The patient is questioned about the presence of pain, paresthesia, and changes in sensation in the distribution of the sciatic nerve, while the needle is being advanced.
- If these symptoms arise, the needle may be in contact with the sciatic nerve and should be repositioned. It is also possible that spasm of the muscle on needle insertion may produce these symptoms and often reproduction of pain occurs with entry into the muscle.
- After negative aspiration, lidocaine (lignocaine) 1% 5 ml is injected.
- Ultrasound may aid placement of the needle (*Fig. 6.4.6 a,b*)

Confirmation of a successful injection

- Relief of pain on abduction of the lower limb against pressure on the lateral knee in the sitting position.

Tips

- If injection is not successful in relieving the pain, it may be repeated at the lateral insertion point. This lies at a

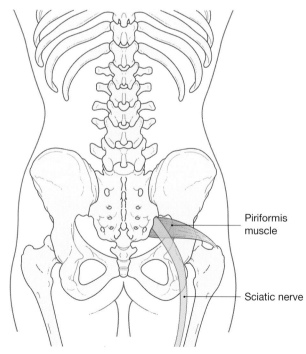

Fig. 6.4.1

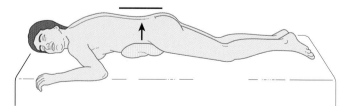

Fig. 6.4.2

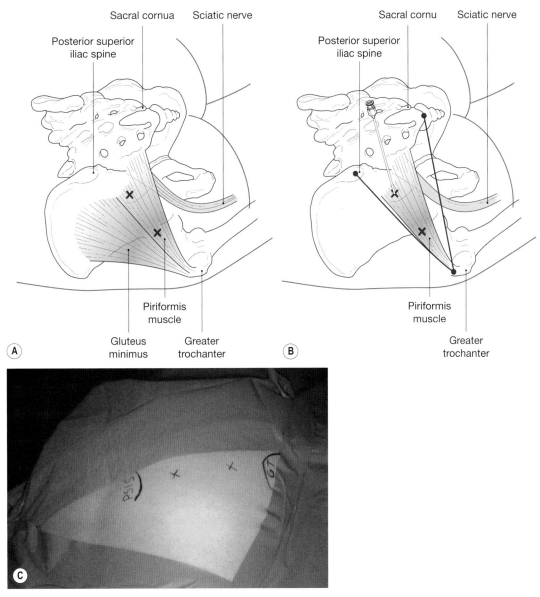

Fig. 6.4.3

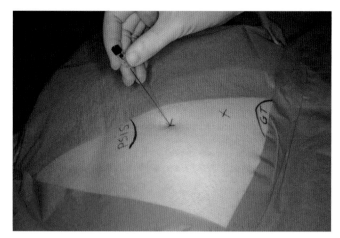

Fig. 6.4.4

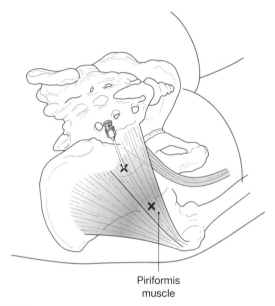

Piriformis
muscle

Fig. 6.4.5

point two-thirds along and 1–3 cm below the line joining the posterior superior iliac spine and the greater trochanter.

Potential problems

• Sciatic nerve block.
• Infection or abscess may occur (rarely).

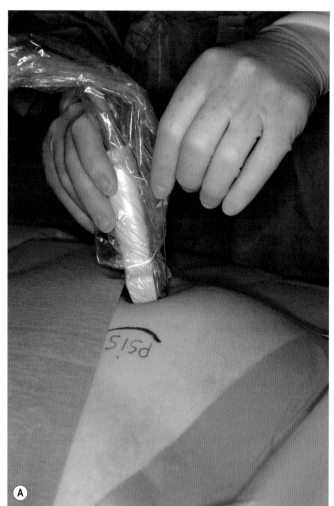

Ⓐ

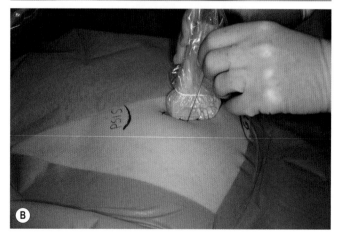

Ⓑ

Fig. 6.4.6

TRANSCUTANEOUS ELECTRICAL NERVE STIMULATION (TENS)

7

Transcutaneous electrical nerve stimulation is thought to modify pain appreciation by stimulation of large fibers thereby blocking (or "closing the gate" to) smaller C-fibers carrying nociceptive impulses. There is also evidence that high-frequency stimulation of the skin increases latency and decreases maximum firing rates in small afferent fibers. This can produce conduction blockade in C-fibers as the current is increased, probably via potassium efflux from the axon. It is thought that a combination of these actions is responsible for the analgesia derived from the use of TENS. This is probably not related to opiate-mediated mechanisms when conventional parameters are used.

Not all pain responds to TENS. If the usual parameters do not produce pain relief, low frequency, high intensity stimulation may be tried. This means that the current amplitude is increased to a level that produces mild discomfort and muscle stimulation. Analgesia from this type of stimulation may be due to opiate-mediated mechanisms. Burst stimulation means short bursts of high frequency stimulation delivered at 1–2 Hz and may also relieve pain that is not responsive to conventional TENS.

A TENS trial may be carried out prior to giving the unit to the patient to use at home. This allows the patient to become familiar with the use of TENS, and to ensure that the pain is not aggravated by its use. A minimum of one hour is recommended as the trial period. This will indicate whether the patient is likely to respond to TENS. However, failure to respond within this time period does not necessarily mean that there will be no response if used for longer periods, or with different settings. It is important to allow the patient to use the TENS at home for a period of at least 14 days.

The TENS stimulator is a battery-operated pulse generator which has several controls. These include an on/off switch plus amplitude control, frequency control, mode selector, and width control. In addition, multichannel units have amplitude controls for each channel. The pulse generator connects to leads that then connect to electrodes, which are applied to the skin. Electrodes are applied in pairs, and are positioned so that they lie along the direction of the nerves in the area being treated, e.g. longitudinally in the limbs, but dermatomally in the trunk.

Control settings (*Figs 7.1.1, 7.1.2*)

CONTINUOUS STIMULATION
- Amplitude set to zero.
- Pulse width set to midrange.
- Switch to continuous mode.
- Increase pulse amplitude level gradually to the maximum level for comfort (sensation should be strong but not painful).
- Adjust pulse frequency to maximum level for comfort (amplitude may be reduced as pulse width is increased).
- Adjust pulse width to maximum level for comfort.
- Maintain for 45–60 minutes.

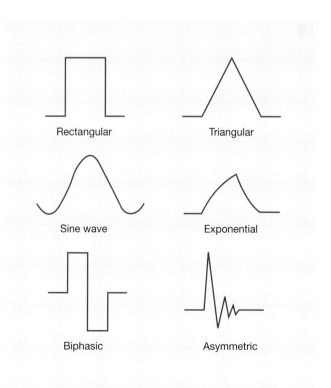

Fig. 7.1.1

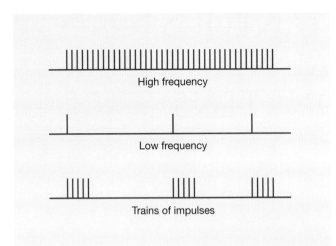

High frequency

Low frequency

Trains of impulses

Fig. 7.1.2

Modulated settings

BURST STIMULATION

- All controls set to zero.
- Switch to pulsed mode.
- Frequency set to 1–2 Hz.
- Increase amplitude and pulse width as with continuous mode described above.
- Maintain for 45–60 minutes.

LOW-FREQUENCY HIGH-INTENSITY STIMULATION

- All controls set to zero.
- Increase amplitude to level where the muscle underlying the electrodes twitches visibly but not painfully.
- Increase frequency to 2–4 Hz.
- Maintain for short period (5–15 minutes).

All the types of stimulation should be tried for each pain, and the effects on the pain should be compared. The optimum parameters must be found by trial and error. The patient is usually advised to begin by using TENS for at least one hour three times a day. Once the effect of TENS on the pain is known it is recommended that stimulation should be discontinued after 30 minutes if the patient experiences one or more hours of analgesia from a single application. If pain relief is achieved only during stimulation, the unit can be kept on constantly. However, electrode sites should be changed every 24 hours. Occasionally, skin rash under the electrodes may occur and this problem may be minimized by frequent rotation of the electrode sites and with topical steroids. However, very few side effects are associated with the use of TENS. Electrical skin burns may occur if TENS is applied to skin with poor innervation and it is necessary to ensure that there is normal sensation prior to applying the electrodes. Allergic reaction to the electrodes or the adhesive tape has also been described, but is not common.

Use of TENS is contraindicated on areas over the anterior neck (stimulation of carotid sinus, larynx), over the pregnant uterus or in the presence of a cardiac pacemaker.

Note: Description of the insertion technique of a spinal cord stimulator or peripheral nerve stimulator is outside the scope of this text as the techniques are specific to the different types of stimulator.

SUGGESTED CORTICOSTEROIDS

Drug name	Duration of action	Equivalent dosage (mg)	Anti-inflammatory potency (relative)	Mineralocorticoid potency (relative)
Triamcinolone[a]	12–36 h	4	5	0
Methylprednisolone	12–36 h	4	5	0.5
Dexamethasone	48 h	0.75	25	0
Hydrocortisone	12 h	20	1	2

[a]Triamcinolone diacetate recommended for central neuroaxial injections.

Corticosteroid injection side effects

LOCAL SIDE EFFECTS
- Atrophy of subcutaneous tissue
- Rupture of injected tendon
- Depigmentation of skin
- Infection

SYSTEMIC SIDE EFFECTS (HIGHER INCIDENCE WITH LARGER DOSES)
- Skin flushing
- Irregularity of the menstrual cycle
- Impaired glucose tolerance
- Osteoporosis
- Muscle wasting and myopathy
- Arthropathy
- Suppression of adrenal function
- Psychologic upset

SUGGESTED NEUROLYTIC AGENTS

- Aqueous phenol 6%.
- Alcohol 100% may be diluted to 50% (pain on injection may be experienced and it is recommended that the nerve is blocked with local anesthetic prior to injection).

3

RECOMMENDED RESUSCITATION DRUGS AND EQUIPMENT

SUGGESTED RESUSCITATION DRUGS

Drug	Suggested dosage (70 kg adult)	Indication
Atropine	0.2–0.4 mg i.v. increments	Bradycardia from vagal dominance
Ephedrine	5–10 mg i.v. increments	Hypotension from sympathetic block
Lidocaine (lignocaine)	50–100 mg i.v. bolus	Ventricular arrhythmias
Midazolam	1–3 mg i.v. increments	Local anesthetic; seizure activity
Diazepam	2.5–5 mg i.v. increments	Local anesthetic; seizure activity
Thiopental (thiopentone)	50–100 mg i.v. increments	Local anesthetic; seizure activity
Succinylcholine	50–100 mg i.v. bolus	Muscle relaxation; airway control

It is also recommended that the full range of drugs required for advanced cardiac life support (ACLS), including pre-filled syringes, be available in the operating room.

Suggested resuscitation equipment

- Oxygen source
- Bag and masks (full range)
- Breathing system for positive pressure ventilation
- Oro- and nasopharangeal airways (full range)
- Laryngoscopes and blades (full range)
- Endotracheal tube stylets and forceps, e.g. Magill's forceps

DERMATOMES

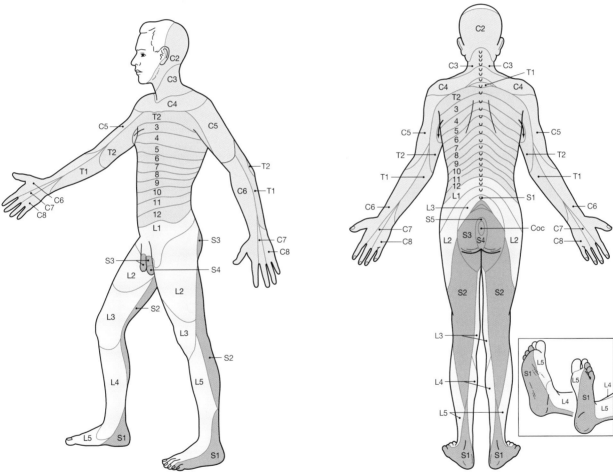

Fig. A.4.1

Fig. A.4.2

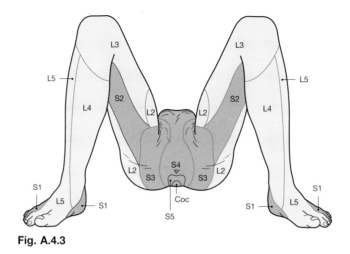

Fig. A.4.3

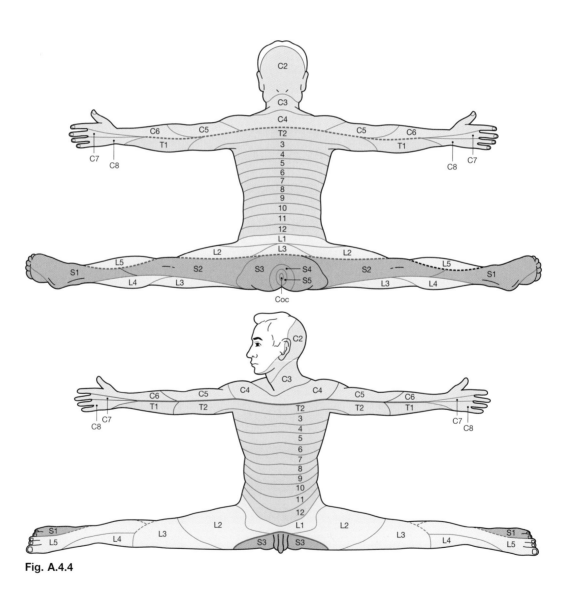

Fig. A.4.4

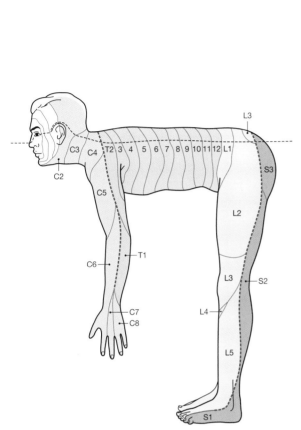

Fig. A.4.5

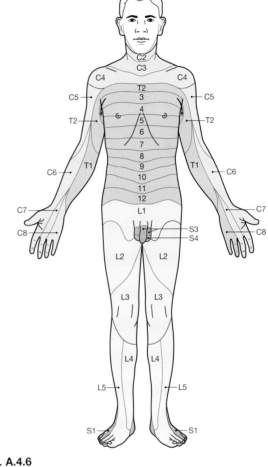

Fig. A.4.6

SPINAL CORD SEGMENTAL MYOTOMES

Each muscle in the body is supplied by a particular level or segment of the spinal cord and by its corresponding spinal nerve.

- C5 also supplies the shoulder muscles and the muscle that we use to bend our elbow.
- C6 is for bending the wrist back.
- C7 is for straightening the elbow.
- C8 bends the fingers.
- T1 spreads the fingers.

- T1–T12 supplies the chest wall and abdominal muscles.
- L2 bends the hip.
- L3 straightens the knee.
- L4 pulls the foot up.
- L5 wiggles the toes.
- S1 pulls the foot down.
- S3, S4 and S5 supply the bladder, bowel and sex organs, and the anal and other pelvic muscles.

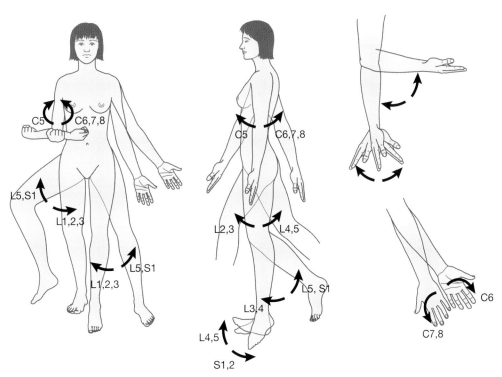

Fig. A.5.1

LUMBO-SACRAL SPINE ANATOMY

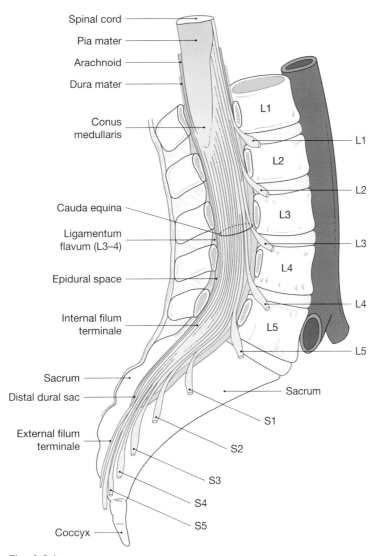

Spinal cord
Pia mater
Arachnoid
Dura mater
Conus medullaris
Cauda equina
Ligamentum flavum (L3–4)
Epidural space
Internal filum terminale
Sacrum
Distal dural sac
External filum terminale
Coccyx

L1
L2
L3
L4
L5

L1
L2
L3
L4
L5

Sacrum
S1
S2
S3
S4
S5

Fig. A.6.1

INDEX

Page numbers followed by "f" indicate figures, "t" indicate tables, and "b" indicate boxes.